AF589520

EMERGENCY ETHICS

Emergency Ethics

Public Health Preparedness and Response

EDITED BY

Bruce Jennings

Center for Humans and Nature &
Vanderbilt University

John D. Arras

University of Virginia

Drue H. Barrett

Centers for Disease Control and
Prevention

Barbara A. Ellis

Centers for Disease Control and
Prevention

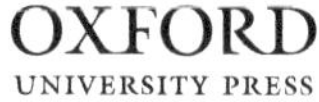

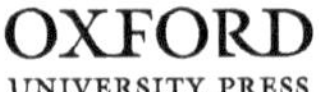

Oxford University Press is a department of the University of Oxford. It furthers the University's objective of excellence in research, scholarship, and education by publishing worldwide.Oxford is a registered trade mark of Oxford University Press in the UK and certain other countries.

Published in the United States of America by Oxford University Press
198 Madison Avenue, New York, NY 10016, United States of America.

First Edition published in 2016

Library of Congress Cataloging-in-Publication Data
Names: Jennings, Bruce, 1949– editor.
Title: Emergency ethics : public health preparedness and response / edited by Bruce Jennings, Center for Humans and Nature & Yale University, John D. Arras, University of Virginia, Drue H. Barrett, Centers for Disease Control and Prevention, Atlanta, Barbara A. Ellis, Centers for Disease Control and Prevention, Atlanta.
Description: New York, NY : Oxford University Press, 2016. | Includes index.
Identifiers: LCCN 2015024090 | ISBN 9780190270742 (hardcover)
Subjects: LCSH: Public health—Moral and ethical aspects. | Emergency medicine—Moral and ethical aspects. | Disaster medicine—Moral and ethical aspects. | Emergency management.
Classification: LCC RA427.25 E44 2016 | DDC 174.2—dc23 LC record available at http://lccn.loc.gov/2015024090

To the Memory of John D. Arras (1945–2015)

philosopher, teacher, and friend

Contents

Preface | ix
Acknowledgments | xi
Contributors | xiii
Introduction | xvii
Barbara A. Ellis, Drue H. Barrett, John D. Arras, and Bruce Jennings

1. Ethical Aspects of Public Health Emergency Preparedness and Response | 1
Bruce Jennings and John D. Arras

2. Justice, Resource Allocation, and Emergency Preparedness: Issues Regarding Stockpiling | 104
Norman Daniels

3. Vulnerable Populations in the Context of Public Health Emergency Preparedness Planning and Response | 135
Madison Powers

4. Public Engagement in Emergency Preparedness and Response: Ethical Perspectives in Public Health Practice | 155
Ruth Gaare Bernheim

5. Professional, Civic, and Personal Obligations in Public Health Emergency Planning and Response | 186
Angus Dawson

6. Research in a Public Health Crisis: The Integrative Approach to Managing the Moral Tensions | 220
Alex John London

INDEX | 263

Preface

BARBARA A. ELLIS, DRUE H. BARRETT,
JOHN D. ARRAS, AND BRUCE JENNINGS

Emergency Ethics: Public Health Preparedness and Response grew out of the work of the Ethics Subcommittee of the Advisory Committee to the Director, Centers for Disease Control and Prevention (CDC). In its examination of the field of all-hazard public health emergency preparedness and response, the Ethics Subcommittee discussed principles and aspects of decision-making in order to provide guidance for public health professionals at all levels engaged in public health emergency planning. To supplement and support the work of the Ethics Subcommittee, the CDC also commissioned five articles on specific topics from leading scholars in bioethics and public health ethics. These original papers, representing the views of the authors, comprise Chapters 2 through 6 of this volume, and we are most grateful to our colleagues Angus Dawson, Norman Daniels, Ruth Gaare Bernheim, Alex John London, and Madison Powers for their work. In addition, a comprehensive white paper, developed by Subcommittee members Bruce Jennings and John D. Arras entitled "Ethical Guidance for Public Health Emergency Preparedness and Response: Highlighting Ethics and Values in a Vital Public Health Service," is available on the CDC website.[1] Chapter 1 of this book is based on the work of that guidance document.

As this book was being prepared for publication, we were saddened by the death of our co-editor and the co-author of Chapter 1, John D. Arras. His efforts informed and improved this work greatly. We are glad it can now be added to his substantial body of published work over a long and distinguished career.

Note

1. http://www.cdc.gov/od/science/integrity/phethics/docs/White_Paper_Final_for_Website_2012_4_6_12_final_for_web_508_compliant.pdf.

Acknowledgments

Emergency Ethics: Public Health Preparedness and Response greatly benefited from a large number of thoughtful public health professionals with wide-ranging experience and expertise. The co-editors gratefully acknowledge the advice and collaboration of the leadership of the Centers for Disease Control and Prevention (CDC), including Richard Besser, Tanja Popovic, and Daniel Sosin.

Ethics Subcommittee members read and commented on drafts of various chapters in this book and provided valuable advice. We thank our Ethic Subcommittee colleagues Ronald Bayer, Georges Benjamin, Vanessa Northington Gamble, Robert Hood, Thomas Hooyman, Nancy E. Kass, Mary desVignes-Kendrick, Barbara Koenig, Kathy Kinlaw, Robert Levine, Bernard Lo, Ruth Macklin, and James Thomas.

We received valuable subject matter expertise from CDC colleagues who formed a Public Health Emergency Preparedness and Response Ethics working group under the CDC Public Health Ethics Committee (PHEC). Members of this working group included May Alston, Drue H. Barrett, Vincent Campbell, Catherine Chow, Marsha Davenport, Barbara A. Ellis, Deborah Esbitt, Roberto Garza, Neelam Ghiya, Brant Goode, Marinda Logan, Charles Magruder, Josephine Malilay, Laura Podewils, Douglas Thoroughman, and Mark T. Wooster.

Moreover, in the course of our research, we were privileged to talk with many people both within the CDC and those working at the state and local levels, in the trenches of emergency preparedness. Their perspective kept us grounded when the ethical analysis tended to become overly abstract. We are grateful to them for giving us their time and the benefit of their experience and expertise. These people included Nelson Arboleda, Steven Boedigheimer, Ralph Bryan, Bruce Burney, Christine Casey, James Cheek, Nathanial Cobb, Steven Coughlin, Roberta Erlwein, David Kennedy, Richard Klomp, Valerie Kokor, Brock Lamont, Lisa M. Lee, Ken Martinez, Elizabeth O'Mara, Bobbie Person, Harald Pietz, Mark White, and the members of the CDC PHEC.

The co-editors and the contributing authors of this book have presented preliminary arguments and findings from the white paper at numerous scholarly and professional conferences, including the National Public Health Preparedness Summit, Association of Practical and Professional Ethics, the American Association of Bioethics and the Humanities, the American Public Health Association, the Protect New York Conference, and the New York State Bar Association Conference on Emergency Planning and the Law. On May 5, 2008, Dr. London organized and sponsored a workshop at Carnegie Mellon University in Pittsburgh to discuss the white paper and the commissioned reports. We are very grateful to the many scholars and public health professionals who attended that meeting and gave us many useful comments and criticisms on that occasion.

Finally, we are grateful to the administrative and research assistance we received from May Alston, Laura Berry, Mariya Deren, Julie DeVries, and Brandon Whitney.

Contributors

John D. Arras, PhD, was the Porterfield Professor of Bioethics, Professor of Philosophy and Public Health Sciences, and core faculty in the Center for Bioethics and Medical Humanities (Medical School) at the University of Virginia. He was a Fellow of the Hastings Center and a member of the US Presidential Commission for the Study of Bioethical Issues.

Drue H. Barrett, PhD, is the lead of the Public Health Ethics Unit within the Office of Scientific Inegrity, Office of the Associate Director for Science, Office of the Director at the US Centers for Disease Control and Prevention (CDC). She also serves as the Chair of the CDC Public Health Ethics Committee. Under her leadership, the CDC has strengthened its infrastructure in public health ethics and established a public health ethics consultation service.

Ruth Gaare Bernheim JD, MPH, is Chair, Department of Public Health Sciences (School of Medicine), and Co-Director, Institute for Practical Ethics and Public Life at the University of Virginia. Her work focuses on integrating ethics in public health practice and education. She has chaired the US Centers for Disease Control and Prevention's Ethics Subcommittee and is currently on the Board of Scientific Counselors, Office of Public Health Preparedness and Response.

Norman Daniels, PhD, is Mary B. Saltonstall Professor in the Department of Global Health and Population at Harvard School of Public Health. His most recent books include *Just Health: Meeting Health Needs Fairly* (Cambridge University Press, 2008) and *Setting Limits Fairly: Learning to Share Resources for Health*, 2nd edition (Oxford University Press, 2008). His research is on justice and health policy, including priority-setting in health systems, fairness and health systems reform, health inequalities, and intergenerational justice.

Angus Dawson, PhD, is Professor of Bioethics and Director of the Centre for Values, Ethics and the Law in Medicine (VELiM) at the University of Sydney, Australia. His main research interests are in public health ethics and research ethics. He is particularly interested in helping policy-makers integrate ethical issues into the work that they do, and he has worked with the World Health Organization, the Public Health Agency of Canada, Public Health England, Médecins Sans Frontières, and the GAVI Alliance.

Barbara A. Ellis, PhD, is the Deputy Director of the Office of Science Quality in the Office of the Associate Director for Science, Office of the Director at the US Centers for Disease Control and Prevention (CDC). She has a diverse professional background and scientific career. Her research interests are focused on zoonotic diseases. She has served the CDC in leadership positions as a senior consultant for cross-agency issues.

Bruce Jennings, MA, is Director of Bioethics at the Center for Humans and Nature and Adjunct Associate Professor at the Vanderbilt University School of Medicine. He has taught public health ethics at the Yale University School of Public Health for many years and is a Fellow and a senior advisor at the Hastings Center, where he served as Executive Director from 1991 to 1999. He is the Editor-in-Chief of the interdisciplinary reference work, *Bioethics, 4th Edition*, 6. vols. (Macmillan Reference USA, 2014). He has written widely on public health ethics and helped to develop

Ethics and Public Health: Model Curriculum with the Association of Schools of Public Health in 2003.

Alex John London, PhD, is Professor of Philosophy and Director of the Center for Ethics and Policy at Carnegie Mellon University. He is an elected Fellow of the Hastings Center and a member of the Working Group on the Revision of the CIOMS 2002 International Ethical Guidelines for Biomedical Research Involving Human Subjects. His work in ethics and research ethics has appeared in *Mind, Science*, and numerous other journals and collections.

Madison Powers, JD, DPhil, is a Senior Research Scholar at the Kennedy Institute of Ethics, and Professor of Philosophy at Georgetown University. He has written widely on normative and practical ethics and is co-author with Ruth Faden of *Social Justice: The Moral Foundations of Public Health and Health Policy* (Oxford University Press, 2006). He was a 1994 recipient of a Robert Wood Johnson Health Policy Investigator Award.

Introduction

BARBARA A. ELLIS, DRUE H. BARRETT,
JOHN D. ARRAS, AND BRUCE JENNINGS

Although the study of ethics as a branch of philosophy has existed for thousands of years, only in the past 40 years has the field of bioethics evolved to address ethical issues specific to public health (Kass, 2001). A code for public health ethics was published in 2002 and has subsequently been adopted by the American Public Health Association (Thomas, Sage, Dillenberg, & Guillory, 2002). However, neither this recent code of ethics nor most scholarly literature on public health ethics directly addresses ethical issues specific to public health emergency preparedness and response. Since September 11, 2001, the field of public health emergency preparedness and response has undergone rapid growth. The need for ethical guidance pertaining to public health emergency preparedness and response has become clear (Larkin & Arnold, 2003), and recommendations regarding development of specific codes of ethics for emergency managers have been proposed (Schneider, 2006).

The purpose of this book is to identify the various ethical principles and values that are germane to public health emergency preparedness and response; to provide guidance on cogent, rigorous processes of ethical reasoning and decision-making in the context of public health emergency preparedness and response; and to propose, where possible, ethical considerations that should inform federal, tribal, state, and local policies, practices, and training as they support local public health emergency preparedness and response efforts.[1]

The Reemergence of Public Health

Public health has been defined as "the science and practice of protecting and improving the overall health of the community through disease prevention and early diagnosis, control of communicable diseases, health education, injury prevention, sanitation, and protection from environmental hazards" (US Department of Homeland Security, 2007). The mission of public health has also been elegantly and simply defined as "fulfilling society's interest in assuring conditions in which people can be healthy" (Institute of Medicine, 1988).

In 1988, the Institute of Medicine called attention to a serious decline in the public health infrastructure of communications, laboratories, surveillance systems, trained personnel, and capacity to respond quickly and adequately to a sudden large-scale threat to population health (Institute of Medicine, 2003). This state of affairs had come about after years of inadequate funding and lack of attention to public health. Ironically, public health was the victim of its own historic successes: vastly improved sanitation, vaccination and the control of infectious diseases, and improvements in air and water quality. The focus of population health, at least in the United States and other developed nations, seemed to be shifting toward the prevention and control of chronic illness and addressing behavioral and lifestyle risk factors. Systems to sustain public health were shifting from traditional public health functions to individual-based clinical care and health insurance coverage to support such care (Lurie, Wasserman, & Nelson, 2006; Rosner & Markovitz, 2006).

The threat of sudden disruption in the health care system and serious danger to life and health on a large scale came to the fore again in the 1990s, as increasing attention was focused on terrorism, spurred by the bombings in a parking garage at the World

Trade Center and at the federal office building in Oklahoma City, as well as the poison gas release in the Tokyo subway system. The 1996, Defense Against Weapons of Mass Destruction Act (P.L. 104–201), commonly known as the Nunn-Lugar-Domenici Act, established a domestic preparedness program and broadened the mandate of the Federal Emergency Management Agency (FEMA) to include attacks by weapons of mass destruction as well as natural disasters. In addition, Congress also passed another significant law, the Antiterrorism and Effective Death Penalty Act of 1996 (P. L. 104–132, Section 511), which provided for additional government controls to deter terrorism. In 1998, the Centers for Disease Control and Prevention (CDC) established the Bioterrorism Preparedness and Response Program, which improved laboratory, surveillance, and emergency response communication capabilities (CDC, 2000). In 1999, Congress charged the Department of Health and Human Services (DHHS) and the CDC with the establishment of a national stockpile of pharmaceuticals and vaccines. In 2000 and early 2001, simulation exercises (TOPOFF 1 and Dark Winter) revealed many remaining shortcomings in emergency preparedness and the ability to respond: poor interagency and intergovernmental communication and coordination, lack of local planning, and inadequate surge capacity (O'Toole, Mair, & Inglesby, 2002).

Such concerns increased exponentially in the aftermath of the terrorist attacks of September 11, 2001, and the use of anthrax as a means of bioterrorism shortly thereafter. Public health emergency preparedness and response was placed squarely at the center of the public health mission and has been a focal point of an infusion of funding, personnel, training, and other resources at the federal, tribal, state, and local levels.

Improvements have been made in many states and locales in their capacity to respond to epidemic or environmental contamination events, but much work remains to be done (Borden, Schmidtlein, Emirch, Piegorsch, & Cutter, 2007; Frickel, 2006; Hearne, Segal, & Earls, 2005; Lister, 2005). Conditions such as West Nile virus, severe acute respiratory syndrome (SARS), multidrug-resistant tuberculosis (MDR-TB), and *Escherichia coli* contamination in the food supply have required public health responses. Some initiatives, such as the national smallpox vaccination plan of 2003, which aimed to immunize the nation's health care workers and first responders, did not succeed because of disagreements over risk–benefit considerations and lack of trust and cooperation among target populations. The devastation of Hurricane Katrina, the destructive earthquake in Haiti, and the earthquake and tsunami in Japan all demonstrated the social and political complexity of emergency planning, response, and recovery (Abbott, 2007; Alexander, 2006; Cooper & Block, 2006; Daniels, Kettl, & Kunreuther, 2006; Hartman & Squires, 2006; Rodriguez & Dynes, 2006; US Department of Justice, 2006; Wachtendorf & Kendra, 2006).

Additional public health challenges loom on the horizon, including avian influenza, possible future instances of bioterrorism, and the prospect of long-term climate change with its multiple threats to public health and well-being (heat waves, flash flooding, violent storms, drought, malnutrition, and large-scale human migration with attendant sanitation and epidemic side effects) (Center for Health and the Global Environment, 2005). These and other threats to the usual systems of disease prevention, health care delivery, and public safety ensure that public health emergency preparedness and response will remain a vital public health responsibility in the 21st century and will be integral to the mission of the CDC and other public health entities.

Some concerns have been raised that public health emergency preparedness and response may narrow the proper focus of public health (Annas, 2002; Annas, Mariner, & Parmet, 2008; Rosner & Markovitz, 2006). This need not be the case. We regard public health emergency preparedness and response as being fully consonant with a broad outlook in public health in which "health" is not simply the absence of disease, but also comprises the conditions and capabilities—material, environmental, social, and political—that enable populations to avoid disease and to experience good health in the context of other elements of well-being and human flourishing (Evans, Marer, & Marmor, 1994). Indeed, in recent years, a consensus has emerged among public health officials and practitioners regarding the appropriate place of public health emergency preparedness and response within public health and its proper scope. This consensus is built around the following points:

- A narrow focus on bioterrorism or weapons of mass destruction is less appropriate than an "all-hazards" approach to planning. Indeed, in 2003, a presidential directive mandated that the US government adopt an all-hazards approach to emergency preparedness and response (US Department of Homeland Security, 2003*a*).
- Preparedness is now understood to encompass more than adequate equipment, deployment of health professionals, training, and supplies. Preparedness also involves the community. A well-prepared community is a community in which the population is medically well-served, a strong public health infrastructure is in place, and community-based public health services are not neglected but are robust and well-integrated into everyday life. If political and budgetary decisions are made that put public health emergency preparedness and response in a zero-sum relationship with other public health programs, such as prenatal and infant nutrition or childhood vaccination programs, it should not be assumed that such decisions genuinely strengthen preparedness.
- A robust, well-functioning infrastructure is necessary for the success of both everyday public health and public health in a time of crisis. Public health emergency preparedness and response and the other aspects of public health supplement, rather than supplant, one another.
- Public trust and confidence are essential in public health emergency preparedness and response, and public health decision-making will be most effective generally when it is transparent and has direct links to the communities it serves.

We embrace these emerging points of agreement and attempt to build on them with the approach to ethics taken in this volume.

Public health emergency preparedness and response goes hand in hand with nonemergency public health policies and programs because a well-funded and thoughtfully designed public health infrastructure is necessary if society is to meet the wide array of currently unforeseeable threats and future disasters. In a similar vein, we believe that the ethical framework for public health generally provides the appropriate framework for public health emergency preparedness and response as well. The moral stakes are high in preparedness activities, but they are also high in ordinary public health practice. Different types of hazards—epidemic, weather-related, environmental, and radiologic—present special circumstances for ethical decision-making and reflection, but they do not require tailor-made ethical principles or values.

Public Health Emergency Preparedness and Response

A public health emergency exists when a situation arises for which the health consequences have the potential to overwhelm routine community capabilities to address them. Although there is no single definition of public health emergency preparedness and response or its scope, it is sufficient for the purposes of this book to begin with the following general notions. Public health emergency preparedness and response involves "the capability of the public health and health-care systems, communities, and individuals, to prevent, protect against, quickly respond to, and recover from health emergencies, particularly those whose scale, timing, or unpredictability threatens to overwhelm routine capabilities" (Nelson, Lurie, Wasserman, & Zakowski, 2007). Moreover, a Presidential Directive defined the term "public health and medical preparedness" as "the existence of plans, procedures, policies, training, and equipment necessary to maximize the ability to prevent, respond to, and recover from major events, including efforts that result in the capability to render an appropriate public health and medical response that will mitigate the effects of illness and injury, limit morbidity and mortality to the maximum extent possible, and sustain societal, economic, and political infrastructure" (US Department of Homeland Security, 2007).

Public health emergency preparedness minimizes the impact of emergencies on affected communities, fosters safe and healthful environments, and ensures sustained public health and medical readiness for communities against disasters or hazards. In addition to terrorism, disasters might include events of other natural and technological origins, including natural epidemics or epizootics of infectious diseases; conventional explosives, toxic chemicals, or radiologic or nuclear devices; industrial or transportation accidents; and climatologic, geologic, or other natural ecologic catastrophes (US Department of Homeland Security, 2008*a*). Thus, to be effective and practical, an all-hazards approach within a multidisciplinary framework must be used by public health in preparedness, response, and recovery activities (National Science and Technology Council, Committee on Environmental and Natural Resources, 2005).

Public health preparedness activities include regulating environmental conditions and food and water safety to minimize disease threats, planning for emergency medical and public health response capabilities, detecting a disease outbreak, conducting epidemiologic investigations to ascertain the nature of a disease epidemic, performing laboratory analyses to inform surveillance and epidemiology, pursuing public health interventions to limit the spread of disease, ensuring the provision of emergency medical treatment and prophylaxis, remediating environmental conditions, and preventing secondary public health emergencies following a disaster (Salinsky, 2002).

Public health emergency preparedness and response is a multidisciplinary endeavor that draws on the traditional bodies of expertise within public health, such as surveillance, epidemiologic analysis, laboratory analysis, and deployment of measures known to be effective in limiting the spread of infection and minimizing human morbidity and mortality. It also draws on the experience and skills of the social and behavioral sciences, risk communication, architecture and planning, environmental science, engineering, and public safety. It must also work together with those responsible for disaster management who come from other fields, and it must negotiate a complicated web of jurisdictional, bureaucratic, and organizational interests and boundaries (de Waal, 2006; Lakoff, 2006; Perrow, 2006; Sturken, 2006). Public health emergency preparedness and response must be cognizant of the legal implications of its functions, and it must work effectively with policy-makers, elected officials, the business community, civic leaders, and the press. It must operate in such a way as to maintain the confidence and trust of the public.

The nature and complexity of the task of public health emergency preparedness and response suggest that it requires ethical analysis at several different levels. First, it falls within the general domain of public health ethics, a field that has developed substantially in recent years (Bayer & Fairchild, 2004; Callahan & Jennings, 2002; Childress et al., 2002; Holland, 2007; Kass, 2001, 2004, 2005; Lappé, 1983, 1986; Mann, 1997; Powers & Faden, 2006; Thomas et al., 2002). Research linking public health ethics explicitly with emergency response has developed slowly. For example, a 2007 review of federal and state influenza pandemic plans showed that, with few exceptions, there was no explicit reference to ethical issues and concepts in these documents (Thomas, Dasgupta, & Martinot, 2007). More recently, however, both at the community level and in academic research, emergency ethics has become a systematic field of study (O'Mathúna, Gordijn, & Clarke, 2014; Zack, 2009).

Preparing for and responding to public health emergencies raises a number of complex ethical issues. Decisions need to be made about allocating scarce resources. Interventions required to protect the public's health may result in limitations on individual freedoms. The professional obligations of public health practitioners may conflict with their personal and family obligations. The public's trust in government recommendations and their perception of the fairness of the planning process may influence the implementation of public health recommendations.

The response to the novel H1N1 influenza virus outbreak and the federal response to Hurricane Katrina have highlighted the need to carefully consider the ethical aspects of public health emergency preparedness and response and to incorporate ethical considerations into emergency planning activities. The articles in this volume fill this gap in the literature of public health ethics and provide analysis and guidance concerning the special area of emergency preparedness and response in public health practice. In the remainder of this introduction, we provide an overview of the CDC's responsibilities for public health emergency preparedness and response, describe the CDC's public health ethics activities, and discuss the genesis and rationale behind the development of this volume.

CDC Responsibilities

The CDC's roles and responsibilities related to public health emergency preparedness and response are mandated by legislation or presidential directives, as well as by policies and directives from DHHS and agency-specific goals and policies. Congressional acts and presidential directives have specifically mandated the need for national-level readiness with respect to emergency preparedness and response. These include the Defense Against Weapons of Mass Destruction Act of 1996 (P. L. 104–201), the Public Health Security and Bioterrorism Preparedness and Response Act of 2002 (P. L. 107–188), the Homeland Security Act of 2002 (P. L. 107–296), the Federal Response Plan and Homeland Security Presidential Directive (HSP)-21 and other HSP directives, and the Pandemic and All-Hazards Preparedness (PAHPA) Act of 2006 (P. L. 109–417).

The National Response Framework (NRF), mandated by the Homeland Security Policy Directive-5, integrates federal domestic prevention, preparedness, response, and recovery into one, all-discipline, all-hazards plan (US Department of Homeland Security, 2003*b*, 2008*b*). The NRF applies to all federal departments and agencies that may be requested to provide assistance in emergencies.

The National Incident Management System (NIMS) is a system used by the NRF to establish a framework for coordination among federal, state, tribal, local, and nongovernmental and private-sector organizations (US Department of Homeland Security, 2008*a*). The roles and responsibilities of the DHHS (and its Operating Divisions, including the CDC) related to emergency preparedness and response activities are consistent with the principles, concepts, terminology, and organizational processes described in the NRF and NIMS. As mandated by PAHPA, the DHHS established the Office of the Assistant Secretary for Preparedness and Response (ASPR). the ASPR is responsible for advising the DHHS Secretary on matters related to public health emergencies and coordinating the activities of federal, state, and local agencies responsible for emergency preparedness (US Department of Health and Human Services, 2007). The primary responsibility for public health emergency preparedness and response resides with state, local, territorial, or tribal governments unless a national emergency has been declared or specific requests for assistance are made to the federal government.

Public Health Ethics at the CDC

In early 2005, the CDC launched a public health ethics initiative to build infrastructure for the analysis of public health ethics issues, such as those raised by public health emergency preparedness and response activities. As part of this initiative, the CDC established an ethics subcommittee under the Advisory Committee to the Director (ACD). This external advisory group was established to provide counsel to the ACD and the CDC Director on a broad range of public health ethics questions and issues arising from programs, scientists, and practitioners and to support CDC in the development of internal capacity to identify, analyze, and resolve ethical issues.

In addition, the CDC formed an internal CDC Public Health Ethics Committee (PHEC). The PHEC is composed of a lead and alternate representative from each of its national centers and representatives from other organizational components within the CDC (e.g., offices within the Office of the Director and science-related workgroups). The mission of the PHEC is to provide leadership in public health ethics at the CDC and to work with CDC staff to integrate the tools of ethical analysis into decisions and day-to-day activities across the CDC.

In September 2006, the CDC requested that the Ethics Subcommittee provide guidance on a comprehensive and systematic approach to ethical issues in public health emergency preparedness and response. The Subcommittee subsequently issued a report, or white paper, on this topic. This report was to expand on another document previously prepared by the subcommittee on ethical considerations for pandemic influenza planning and response. The previous report, *Ethical Guidelines in Pandemic Influenza* (Kinlaw, Barrett, & Levine, 2009), includes a discussion of general ethical considerations as well as specific ethical issues relating to vaccine and antiviral drug distribution and development of interventions that would limit individual freedoms for the protection of the public good. The pandemic influenza guidelines were not intended to provide a comprehensive view of the ethical principles and considerations that public health officials should consider in all emergency preparedness and response activities.

Two Ethics Subcommittee members (John D. Arras, University of Virginia, and Bruce Jennings, Center for Humans and Nature and Yale University) took the lead on developing more comprehensive guidelines. The resulting document, *Ethical Guidance for Public Health Emergency Preparedness and Response: Highlighting Ethics and Values in a Vital Public Health Service*, was presented and discussed in public meetings of the Ethics Subcommittee, was approved by the Ethics Subcommittee in September 2008, and was reviewed and approved by the ACD in October 2008. Subject matter expertise was provided by members of the CDC PHEC Emergency Preparedness and Response Workgroup.[2]

Aims of this Volume

This volume comprises six chapters. The first chapter, by Jennings and Arras, argues that public health emergency preparedness is a distinctive component of public health policy and practice more generally and should be understood as a form of what they call "civic practice" in order to bring the value components and ethical goals of this domain of public health into clear focus. The chapters by Daniels, Powers, Bernheim, Dawson, and London are designed to focus particular attention on core ethical problems in the public health emergency preparedness and response field—ethical use of limited resources, the special needs of vulnerable populations, special obligations of professionals, community involvement in preparedness, and research ethics in emergency situations. The overarching purpose of the volume is to identify ethical principles and values relevant to public health emergency preparedness and response (taking an all-hazards approach) and to reflect on how these values can be integrated into public health decision-making, policy, and practice.

In Chapter 1, Jennings and Arras offer an overview of emergency ethics and a distinctive perspective on emergency preparedness and planning and the ethical public health mission. Their civic practice perspective views emergency preparedness as a form of community engagement and capacity building rather than as simply a public health service provided by trained experts to passive clients. This viewpoint opens up such questions as: What self-consciousness of role, responsibility, and quality performance ought planners adopt? Is emergency planning and response a truly "public" health undertaking, and, if so, how should its public or civic ends be understood? How does this perspective guide us in ethically assessing not only the content of an emergency plan, but also the process through which it is derived? They address general difficult ethical challenges such as the careful and ethically justified restriction on personal liberty and ways of protecting equity and fairness in the distribution of inherently scarce resources and in the distribution of risk and benefit.

In Chapter 2, Norman Daniels argues that health is of special ethical importance because of its contribution to the range of opportunities open to people. Because justice requires equality of opportunity, policy-makers have an obligation to promote population health and to sustain institutions that distribute health benefits fairly. An ethical tension exists between the goal of health maximization and health equity (the "best outcomes vs. fair chances" problem), and Daniels uses the example of stockpiling medical resources in the context of public health emergency preparedness. He points out that, during a public health emergency, reasonable people will disagree about how to reconcile concerns about maximizing aggregate health with concerns about distributing that health fairly. He argues that no available ethical theory or general principles of justice will resolve the tension between best outcomes and fair chances. In the face of that dilemma, public health preparedness policy and planning should rely on a fair, deliberative process that emphasizes accountability for reasonableness. Daniels offers an analysis of four general conditions for ensuring a fair process—publicity, relevance, revisability, and enforcement.

In Chapter 3, Madison Powers describes several kinds of vulnerability to harm that arise in the context of emergency preparedness planning and response policy. First, it should be recognized that there are multiple forms of vulnerability, both medical and socioeconomic, to greater than average harms, and that harms of one kind among some of the most vulnerable populations can magnify and compound harms of other kinds produced by disasters. Second, policy-makers have a duty to identify and anticipate the groups most vulnerable to the greatest magnitude of harm in a disaster, take steps to mitigate that harm in advance of a disaster, and ameliorate predictable harms to vulnerable populations after a disaster.

In Chapter 4, Ruth Gaare Bernheim argues that public engagement plays a necessary and central role in the emergency preparedness and response activities in public health practice. Like public health practice in general, public health emergency preparedness is both a political and social undertaking. In a liberal democracy, public engagement in public health emergency preparedness is required as a fundamental feature of governance to assure that government authority and government actions have political legitimacy. Public engagement is also essential for the social practices and activities of emergency preparedness, which provide a foundation for public health professional and community relationships and for public trust. The primary role for public engagement in public health emergency preparedness is grounded in a number of ethical principles, such as fairness and respect for the rights of individuals in a community, which animate the practice of public health and are enumerated in the *Principles of the Ethical Practice of Public Health* (See Table 4.1, p. 165). Public engagement should take place in at least two ways: first, through deliberation about the fundamental societal values and tensions at stake in public health emergency preparedness, and, second, through consultation, which provides for the two-way exchange of information and views about specific emergency preparedness and response services in a particular community, ranging from data collection and needs assessment to program planning and evaluation. Ethical principles and values can help to frame the goals, methods, and outcome measures of these forms of public engagement in public health emergency preparedness. Systematic evaluation of different approaches is needed to establish best practices. As both government authorities and the providers of essential public health services, public health officials have the responsibility to actively seek and provide opportunities for public engagement as part of a deliberative, evidence-based process of decision-making for public health emergency preparedness.

In Chapter 5, Angus Dawson explores the responsibilities associated with public health emergency planning and response. He finds that these responsibilities form a complex web of prima facie moral obligations. These obligations can be categorized and a taxonomy developed based on how they come into existence. However, such a taxonomy does not provide any justification for seeing certain kinds of obligations as always taking priority over others. Indeed, we cannot say before the fact which particular obligation ought to take priority in reference to an actual situation. In considering the more practical issue of the conflicting obligations faced by health professionals in public health emergency preparedness situations, role obligations—particularly the duty of care—are of major importance. Published empirical evidence from emergency instances, particularly the recent experience with the outbreak of SARS, supports the discussion and conclusions regarding the moral obligations of public health professionals. A general framework for thinking about moral obligations relevant to emergency preparedness can aid in understanding the core obligations of public health providers, and articulating some empirically informed discussion of actual cases can serve as a means of ensuring that we do not focus too much on ideal obligations.

The volume concludes with Alex John London's discussion of the profound moral tensions that can arise from the conduct of research in the context of a public health emergency. In Chapter 6, London argues that two of the leading frameworks for assessing the risks, benefits, and social value of clinical research—the concept of equipoise and the duty not to exploit persons—have important shortcomings that limit their usefulness in this context. An alternative, which he calls the "integrative approach," holds out promise for resolving these tensions because it is a framework for evaluating public health emergency research that derives operationally useful practical guidance from a compelling normative foundation. London's chapter describes various frameworks for assessing research in the context of a public health emergency and explains how the integrative approach can fulfill the social mission of providing practical guidance to decision-makers who may embrace diverse and divergent life plans.

The chapters collected in this volume offer a diverse and comprehensive analysis of the ethical considerations facing emergency planning, response, and recovery. It is intended to be a resource for public health practitioners and policy-makers as well as a work of interest to scholars and students in the fields of public health ethics and bioethics. Both government officials and citizen groups must recognize basic ethical tenets and considerations, integrate these concepts into their planning, and institutionalize procedures that address considerations of liberty, equity, and community resilience. In the final analysis, ethical decision-making and public trust are the necessary foundation of all viable public health preparedness and response efforts.

Notes

1. There is no short term in use to refer to the activities we focus on in this volume. We will be concerned with the public health dimension of emergency planning and not so much with law enforcement and public safety dimensions, although we recognize that the boundaries may be often indistinct and overlapping. We also intend the term to cover pre-event planning and preparation, event response, and post-event recovery.

2. Members of the CDC PHEC Emergency Preparedness and Response Workgroup included May Alston, Drue H. Barrett, Vincent Campbell, Catherine Chow, Marsha Davenport, Barbara A. Ellis, Deborah Esbitt, Roberto Garza, Neelam Ghiya, Brant Goode, Marinda Logan, Charles Magruder, Josephine Malilay, Laura Podewils, Douglas Thoroughman, and Mark T. Wooster.

References

Abbott, E. B. (2007). Book review of disaster: Hurricane Katrina and the failure of homeland security. *Journal of Homeland Security and Emergency Management*, *4*, published online 2007-03-21.

Alexander, D. (2006). Symbolic and practical interpretations of the Hurricane Katrina disaster in New Orleans. In *Understanding Katrina: Perspectives from the social sciences*. Social Science Research Council. Available at http://understandingkatrina.ssrc.org/Alexander/.

Annas, G. J. (2002). Bioterrorism, public health, and civil liberties. *New England Journal of Medicine*, *346*, 1337–1342.

Annas, G. J., Mariner, W. K., & Parmet, W. E. (2008). *Pandemic preparedness: The need for a public health–not a law enforcement/*

national security approach. New York: American Civil Liberties Union. Available at http://www.aclu.org/privacy/medical/33642pub20080114.html.

Antiterrorism and Effective Death Penalty Act of 1996. Section 511. Enhanced penalties and control of biologic agents. Public Law 104–132 (April 24, 1996).

Bayer, R., & Fairchild, A. L. (2004). The genesis of public health ethics. *Bioethics*, *18*, 473–492.

Borden, K. A., Schmidtlein, M. C., Emirch, C. T., Piegorsch, W. W., & Cutter, S. L. (2007). Vulnerability of U.S. cities to environmental hazards. *Journal of Homeland Security and Emergency Management*, *4*, published online 2007-06-27.

Callahan, D., & Jennings, B. (2002). Ethics and public health: Forging a strong relationship. *American Journal of Public Health*, *92*, 169–176.

Center for Health and the Global Environment. (2005). *Climate change futures: Health, ecological and economic dimensions*. Boston: Harvard Medical School. Available at http://coralreef.noaa.gov/aboutcrcp/strategy/reprioritization/wgroups/resources/climate/resources/cc_futures.pdf.

Centers for Disease Control and Prevention (CDC). (2000). Biological and chemical terrorism: Strategic plan for preparedness and response. Recommendations of the CDC Strategic Planning Workgroup. *MMWR*, *49* (RR-04), 1–14.

Childress, J. F., Faden, R. R., Gaare, R. D., Gostin, L. O., Kahn, J., Bonnie, R. J., . . . Nieburg, P. (2002). Public health ethics: Mapping the terrain. *Journal of Law, Medicine & Ethics*, *30*, 170–178.

Cooper, C., & Block, R. (2006). *Disaster: Hurricane Katrina and the failure of homeland security*. New York: Times Books.

Daniels, N., Kettl, D. F., & Kunreuther, H. (2006). *On risk and disaster: Lessons from Hurricane Katrina*. Philadelphia, PA: University of Philadelphia Press.

de Waal, A. (2006). An imperfect storm: Narratives of calamity in a liberal-technocratic age. In *Understanding Katrina: Perspectives from the Social Sciences*. Social Science Research Council. Available at http://understandingkatrina.ssrc.org/deWaal/.

Defense Against Weapons of Mass Destruction Act of 1996 (Public Law 104–201, Title XIV) (September 23, 1996).

Evans, R. G., Marer, M. L., & Marmor, T. R. (1994). *Why are some people healthy and others not?* New York: Aldine de Gruyter.

Frickel, S. (2006). Our toxic gumbo: Recipe for a politics of environmental knowledge. In *Understanding Katrina: Perspectives from the Social Sciences*. Social Science Research Council. Available at http://understandingkatrina.ssrc.org/Frickel/.

Hartman, C., & Squires, G. D. (2006). *There is no such thing as a natural disaster: Race, class, and Hurricane Katrina*. New York: Routledge.

Hearne, S. A., Segal, L. M., & Earls, M. J. (2005). *Ready or not? Protecting the public's health from disease, disasters, and bioterrorism*. Washington, DC: Trust for America's Health.

Holland, S. (2007). *Public health ethics*. Cambridge: Polity Press.

Homeland Security Act of 2002 (Public Law 107–296) (November 25, 2002).

Institute of Medicine. (1988). *The future of public health*. Washington, DC: National Academies Press.

Institute of Medicine. (2003). *The future of the public's health in the 21st century*. Washington, DC: National Academies Press.

Kass, N. (2001). An ethics framework for public health. *American Journal of Public Health*, *91*, 1776–1782.

Kass, N. (2005). An ethics framework for public health and avian influenza pandemic preparedness. *Yale Journal of Biology and Medicine*, *78*, 239–254.

Kass, N. E. (2004). Public health ethics: From foundations and frameworks to justice and global public health. *Journal of Law, Medicine & Ethics*, *32*, 232–242.

Kinlaw, K., Barrett D. H., & Levine R. J. (2009). Ethical guidelines in pandemic influenza: Recommendations of the Ethics Subcommittee of the Advisory Committee of the Director, Centers for Disease Control and Prevention. *Disaster Medicine and Public Health Preparedness*, *3*(Suppl 2), 1–8.

Lakoff, A. (2006). From disaster to catastrophe: The limits of preparedness. In *Understanding Katrina: Perspectives from the social sciences*. Social Science Research Council. Available at http://understandingkatrina.ssrc.org/Lakoff/.

Lappé, M. (1983). Values and public health: Value considerations in setting health policy. *Theoretical Medicine*, *4*, 71–92.

Lappé, M. (1986). Ethics and public health. In J. M. Last (Ed.), *Public health and preventive medicine* (12th ed., pp. 1867–1877). Norwalk, CT: Appleton-Century-Crofts.

Larkin, G. L., & Arnold, J. (2003). Ethical considerations in emergency planning, preparedness, and response to acts of terrorism. *Prehospital Disaster Medicine, 18*, 170–178.

Lister, S. A. (2005). *An overview of the US public health system in the context of emergency preparedness.* CRS Report for Congress. Washington, DC: Congressional Research Service, Library of Congress.

Lurie, N., Wasserman, J., & Nelson C. D. (2006). Public health preparedness: Evolution or revolution? *Health Affairs, 25*, 935–945.

Mann, J. M. (1997). Medicine and public health, ethics and human rights. *Hastings Center Report, 27*, 6–13.

National Science and Technology Council, Committee on Environment and Natural Resources. (2005). *Grand challenges for disaster reduction.* A report of the Subcommittee on Disaster Reduction. Available at http://www.sdr.gov/docs/SDRGrandChallengesforDisasterReduction.pdf.

Nelson, C., Lurie, N., Wasserman, J., & Zakowski, S. (2007). Conceptualizing and defining public health emergency preparedness. *American Journal of Public Health, 97*(Suppl 1), S9–S11.

O'Mathúna, D. P., Gordijn, B., & Clarke, M. (Eds.). (2014). *Disaster bioethics: Normative issues when nothing is normal.* Dordrecht: Springer Press.

O'Toole, T., Mair, M., & Inglesby, T. V. (2002). Shining light on "Dark Winter." *Clinical Infectious Diseases, 34*, 972–983.

Pandemic and All-Hazards Preparedness Act of 2006 (Pubic Law No. 109–417) (December 19, 2006).

Perrow, C. (2006). Using organizations: The case of FEMA. In *Understanding Katrina: Perspectives from the social sciences.* Social Science Research Council. Available at http://understandingkatrina.ssrc.org/Perrow/.

Powers, M., & Faden, R. (2006). *Social justice: The moral foundations of public health and health policy.* Oxford: Oxford University Press.

Public Health Security and Bioterrorism Preparedness and Response Act of 2002 (Public Law 107–88) (June 12, 2002).

Rodriguez, H., & Dynes, R. (2006). Finding and framing Katrina: The social construction of disaster. In *Understanding Katrina: Perspectives from the social sciences.* Social Science

Research Council. Available at http://understandingkatrina.ssrc.org/Dynes_Rodriguez/.

Rosner, D., & Markovitz, G. (2006). *Are we ready? Public health since 9/11*. Berkeley: University of California Press.

Salinsky, E. (2002). *Public health emergency preparedness: Fundamentals of the system*. Washington, DC: George Washington University Press.

Schneider, R. O. (2006). Principles of ethics for emergency managers. *Journal of Emergency Management, 4*, 56–62.

Sturken, M. (2006). Weather media and homeland security: Selling preparedness in a volatile world. In *Understanding Katrina: Perspectives from the social sciences*. Social Science Research Council. Available at http://understandingkatrina.ssrc.org/Sturken/.

Thomas, J. C., Dasgupta, N., & Martinot, A. (2007). Ethics in a pandemic: A survey of the state pandemic influenza plans. *American Journal of Public Health, 97*(Suppl 1), S26–S31.

Thomas, J. C., Sage, M., Dillenberg, J., & Guillory, V. J. (2002). A code of ethics for public health. *American Journal of Public Health, 92*, 1057–1059.

US Department of Health and Human Services. (2007). *Assistant Secretary for Preparedness and Response. Strategic plan, 2007–2012. "A nation prepared."* Available at https://www.hsdl.org/?view&did=33528.

US Department of Homeland Security. (2003a). Homeland Security Presidential Directive (HSPD)-8. Available at http://www.fas.org/irp/offdocs/nspd/hspd-8.html.

US Department of Homeland Security. (2003b). *Presidential Directive/HSPD-5: Management of domestic incidents*. Washington, DC: Executive Office of the President.

US Department of Homeland Security. (2007). *Presidential Directive/HSPD-21: Public health and medical preparedness*. Washington, DC: Executive Office of the President.

US Department of Homeland Security. (2008a). *National incident management system*. Available at http://www.fema.gov/pdf/emergency/nims/NIMS_core.pdf.

US Department of Homeland Security. (2008b). *National response framework*. Available at: http://www.fema.gov/pdf/emergency/nrf/nrf-core.pdf.

US Department of Justice. (2006). *Making community emergency preparedness and response programs accessible to people with disabilities*. Available at http://www.ada.gov/emergencyprep.htm.

Wachtendorf, T., & Kendra, J. M. (2006). Improvising disaster in the city of jazz: Organizational response to Hurricane Katrina. In *Understanding Katrina: Perspectives from the social sciences*. Social Science Research Council. Available at http://understandingkatrina.ssrc.org/Wachtendorf_Kendra/.

Zack, N. (2009). *Ethics for disaster.* Lanham, MD: Rowman and Littlefield.

1

Ethical Aspects of Public Health Emergency Preparedness and Response

BRUCE JENNINGS AND JOHN D. ARRAS

All partners who can contribute to action as a public health system should be encouraged to assess their roles and responsibilities, consider changes, and devise ways to better collaborate with other partners. They can transform the way they "do business" to better act to achieve a healthy population on their own and position themselves to be part of an effective partnership in assuring the health of the population.

Institute of Medicine (2003)

Introduction

Our aim in this chapter is to provide an orientation for the future exploration of ethical issues in public health emergency preparedness and response (hereafter referred to simply as "emergency preparedness"). Much work has been done in the past decade on specific ethical issues that arise in the context of certain facets of emergency preparedness, such as the ethics of allocating scarce resources like vaccines or emergency equipment, and the ethical issues that arise in relationship to infectious disease, such as influenza (Annas, Mariner, & Parmet, 2008; Battin, Francis, Jacobson, & Smith, 2009; DeBruin et al., 2010; Garrett, Vawter, Prehn, DeBruin, & Gervais, 2008; Kinlaw, Barrett, & Levine, 2009; Meslin, Alyea, & Helft, 2007; University of Toronto Joint Centre for

Bioethics, 2005; Vawter, Gervais, & Garrett, 2008; Verweij, 2006; World Health Organization, 2007). In addition, a significant social scientific literature exists on factors concerning the response and recovery of social systems to crisis situations. These sociological theories and empirical studies certainly have value implications, but they rarely engage in explicit ethical analysis.[1]

The aim of this chapter is to consider what kind of activity public health emergency preparedness as a whole is and to ask what ethical goals should orient an activity of that kind (Zack, 2009). More specifically, we identify a particular perspective from which to view the complexity of emergency preparedness, and that perspective involves seeing emergency preparedness as a civic practice. The notion of a "practice" is a special term of art in philosophical and social scientific studies of purposeful human agency (MacIntyre, 2007; Schön, 1984; Schön & Rein, 1997). It refers to a complex form of social activity that is systematic, rule-governed, and has definable inherent values. A practice can be said to achieve (or fail to achieve) instrumentally certain social goods external to it, and, in its pursuit of those external objectives, the practice can also realize (or fail to realize) its own internal or inherent values. A practice can be either private or public, individualistic or civic. A "civic practice" is one that pertains to and affects not only the rights and interests of private individuals, but also the common good: the values and obligations of the community as a whole. Manifestly, public health emergency preparedness has societal as well as individual significance and is a civic rather than a private form of practice. Preparedness is something that citizens enact, not something that individuals purchase and consume.

In this analysis, we single out for special discussion seven social goods (beneficial objectives) that constitute ethical goals of public health emergency preparedness as a civic practice. These are goals that we believe are pertinent to an ethical evaluation of how the practice of emergency preparedness should be conducted regardless of the specific type of hazard or emergency in question.

As research on public health ethics and on the ethics of various areas of emergency preparedness develops, it is becoming standard to identify and embrace variously described "frameworks" of ethical principles or standards. We do not follow this approach in this chapter. The norms and values—the ethical goals and social goods—we analyze are not general moral rules or imperatives that are designed to produce a certain outcome or to arrive ethically at a particular destination: the right answer or the right action. Instead of focusing on the right destination, these goals and goods focus on the appropriate ethical orientation. They concern not so much the end points, but the compass points of ethical emergency preparedness. We also intend to pay attention to certain domains, such as community capacity and resilience, community participation, civic responsibility, and public trust. These topics are of central importance to emergency preparedness, but, although they are often addressed from an explanatory social scientific perspective, they have not been adequately addressed from an explicitly ethical or normative point of view.

In sum, we focus not on abstractly conceived ethical principles, but on ethical goals or social goods that should be understood in reference to the distinctive type of practice that emergency preparedness planning constitutes. In many ethical analyses in the field of bioethics, abstract, general principles are applied to specific situations or cases that are often treated as static snapshots of decision-making rather than as an ongoing narrative or drama unfolding, often surprisingly, over time. However, analysis based on general ethical principles rarely provides practical guidance for public health practitioners immersed in an emergency response in which decisions must be made quickly amid quickly evolving information and circumstances. In light of this, it is all the more important to grasp emergency preparedness as a dynamic activity, a form of practice with external goals and inherent values.

This enables us to do two things. First, it provides an ethical conception of emergency preparedness as a whole, brought about by the coordination of many groups, disciplines, and interests and drawing on numerous bodies of knowledge and expertise. This is a study of what may be called the *ethics of* emergency preparedness; that is, an account of its moral point and human value, an account of why it is an activity that should be engaged in at all. Second, it opens the door to an exploration of what might be called the *ethics in* emergency preparedness; that is, the specific moral dilemmas, choices, and quandaries that arise in the course of actually doing emergency preparedness. It addresses particular aspects of preparedness and response plans and specific decisions that planners and communities have to make that require balancing many diverse and sometimes conflicting values.

This chapter has nine sections. We begin with a brief reflection on why an ethical perspective is crucial in emergency preparedness. We then offer a commentary on the main ethical goals and social goods of emergency preparedness. Subsequent sections address the protection of life and health, the value of individual liberty and ethical justifications for its restriction in the context of emergency preparedness, justice and preparedness, ethical responsibilities toward persons and groups with special vulnerability, communication and civic participation, professional obligations and divided loyalties for health professionals, and civic responsibility or emergency citizenship. Finally, we offer some recommendations on reasonable decision-making in emergency preparedness planning and response. Many of these issues are analyzed in greater detail by other authors in subsequent chapters of this book.

Why Ethics Matters

In order to reduce disease and promote health, public health must be an agent of change—behavioral change among individuals and institutional change in societies. Such change is never easy, even when unusual loss of life, injury, severe illness, and social disruption are threatened. Existing patterns of individual behavior and social institutions are embedded in structures of power and in social expectations and cultural norms. Behavioral and institutional change, no matter how seemingly urgent and reasonable, still requires ethical justification. This is because the principal goals of public health—security, safety, health, and well-being—must be balanced with other important values. Ethical justification is also required for emergency public health measures because, for the most part, public health and public safety authorities must rely on voluntary compliance by large numbers of people, and voluntary behavior change in turn depends on the fact that people see good reasons for their compliance, including good ethical reasons.

Ethical reasoning and sensitivity is always important in public health, but it is especially important in the sensitive and complex area of public health emergency preparedness. Indeed, the requirements of ethical justification in the context of emergency preparedness are quite demanding, and the ethical stakes are high because changes required are often disruptive and momentous, they may be financially costly, and they usually involve some form of state action. They involve the creation of legal sanctions and enforcement, the creation of administrative structures, the investment and allocation of resources, and the mobilization of popular support (Hanfling, Altevogt, Viswanathan, & Gostin, 2012; O'Mathúna, Gordijn, & Clarke, 2014).

When considering ethics in emergency preparedness, decision-making with incomplete or imperfect knowledge and under pressure of time is one of the central concerns. Sound factual information is one foundation for ethically justified decision-making. Careful, thorough, and deliberate assessment of options is another. In the real world of emergency response, and even in the less pressured situation of prior emergency preparedness planning, both of these prerequisites of ethical decision-making may be compromised. But plans must be drawn, decisions and actions must be taken nonetheless (Knobler, Mack, Mahmoud, & Lemon, 2004*a*).

To be sure, facts in and of themselves rarely drive or compel decisions because factual information requires assessment and evaluation, and judgments of value inevitably enter into the interpretation of facts and their meaning (Smith, 2013). "Judgment," as we use it here, is a general term covering such things as assessment, estimation of risk and probability, conjecture, understanding of human motivation and behavior, sensitivity to cultural or symbolic meaning, discernment, taste, a sense of propriety, and the tacit knowledge ("intuition") that comes from experience (Schön & Rein, 1997). Without judgment, facts are of limited use and provide little guidance. If public health planning without facts is like sailing in a fog, planning without judgment is like sailing without a rudder.

In describing and analyzing facts, the notion of special training and expertise has an obvious application, and it can be strong enough to warrant granting special power and authority to those who possess it. In matters of judgment, however, the notion of expertise as the possession of a small and definable group of persons is much more dubious. This means that public health planning is always a compound of expertise and common sense—trained analytical knowledge and knowledge gained from experience; technical science and "street science" (Corburn, 2005; Fain, Viswanathan, & Altevogt, 2012; Scarry, 2011; Wizemann, Reeve, & Altevogt, 2013*a*). This is one of the reasons for embracing the civic model of the practice of emergency preparedness rather than the consumerist model. Emergency preparedness has an impact not only on the health and safety of individuals, but also on their liberty, autonomy, civil and human rights, property, and other fundamental interests. Emergency preparedness planning must face the occasional necessity of directing people to behave in a certain way during an emergency to protect the health interests of the population and to promote their own best interests, even if they are inclined to behave in other ways.

"Paternalism" is the term used to convey the notion of a restriction of an individual's freedom of choice for the sake of protecting or promoting that individual's best interests. Emergency preparedness is inherently prone to paternalism because one of its basic missions is to guide behavior during an emergency in such a way that long-term interests prevail over short-term interests. The inclination of many people will be to resist the actions that sound emergency preparedness calls for and to behave with other ends in view. People may want to be together with others during an outbreak of infectious disease when they should isolate themselves. They may want to leave their homes and flee when they would be safer, and emergency efforts would be more effective, if they stayed off the roads. Or some may want to stay home, which feels safe and familiar, in order to protect their belongings or their pets when the safest course is to evacuate. People may seek medicines that are inappropriate for them to take or unjust for them to hoard. They may act on the basis of rumor, unreliable or false information, or on the basis of irrational thinking concerning risk. Emergency preparedness must foresee these understandable but nonetheless counterproductive behaviors, and it must somehow prevent or at least discourage them.

These unavoidable paternalistic aspects of emergency preparedness alone would be enough to make it a subject warranting close ethical attention. American culture has strongly anti-paternalistic currents within it. Americans value individual freedom of choice and self-reliance. They are suspicious of authority, not deferential to it or cowed by it. In the past generation, the American public has come to the point where it no longer believes that "father knows best," much less that doctor knows best, and even less that health commissioner knows best. In addition, many Americans are skeptical of uses of power that claim to be in the best interests of the powerless or in the public interest but all too often seem to serve the interests of the powerful.

This is not to say that during an emergency most people will not comply with emergency regulations and directives; that they will not turn to their leaders, experts, and other authorities for protection and guidance; or that they will not be willing to forgo significant personal liberty in return for a promise of greater protection and safety. When their community is threatened, people even in a privacy-oriented and individualistic culture will volunteer, feel a sense of solidarity, and make sacrifices for each other and for the common good (Keystone Center, 2007; King's Fund, 2004; Solnit, 2009). However, the individualism of American culture, reinforced by ethical systems that stress autonomy, rights, and civil liberties, will have an impact, especially on the planning and recovery phases of emergency preparedness. In the planning phase, directives that restrict liberty must be fully explained and justified. In the aftermath or recovery phase of a public health emergency, experience shows that solidarity and self-sacrifice often give way to disillusionment, recrimination, and even litigation. It is probably in the nature of any emergency plan that it cannot protect (or please) all of the people all of the time. To offset this, it is important to have ongoing monitoring of the use of authority and power during the implementation of emergency plans. This is to ensure that power and authority are not abused ("Who watches the guardians?") and that coercive measures were justified under the circumstances. Ongoing and post-crisis evaluation and assessment are also important to gauge the effectiveness of emergency plans, to learn from mistakes, and to make improvements for the future.

Throughout this chapter, we argue in favor of public health approaches that employ the least restrictive alternatives, community involvement, and transparent communication. Nonetheless, the use of coercion and secrecy—or deliberately withholding information from the public—although they should be avoided if possible and as a general rule cannot be morally ruled out categorically. Their ethical justification in particular instances will be a matter of context and circumstance (Conly, 2013; Gaylin & Jennings, 2003). Mandatory evacuation measures or quarantine may be unavoidable and ethically justified under extreme circumstances. Withholding information from the public may be necessary in order to prevent panic and counterproductive behavior on a large scale. It is precisely because measures may be taken in emergencies that would ordinarily be unacceptable in normal times that it is so important that public health planners not wait for disaster to strike before trying to work out a viable scheme of priorities (Knobler et al., 2004*b*). The role of ethics in the planning phase before a crisis, as in the recovery phase afterward, is to define reasonably just, humane, and responsible parameters for action and decision-making. Even within those parameters, there is no way to ensure that moral mistakes will not be made, but emergency planners and responders must always be prepared to be accountable for their conduct in terms of the good reasons that they had for deciding and acting as they did (Walzer, 1973).

Two Understandings of Emergency Preparedness: Civic and Consumerist

Aside from the fact that public health emergencies may require some paternalistic measures, a more fundamental question arises about the civic and democratic implications of emergency response. There is a tendency to see emergencies as requiring the centralization of top-down authority and to see emergency preparedness as outside normal democratic governance. The so-called *emergency exception* is the legal suspension of the rule of law (Agamben, 2005; Bröckling, Krasmann, & Lemke, 2010). However, this authoritarian command model of decision-making both underestimates the capacity for responsible conduct and social coordination that exists in nonemergency periods, and it exaggerates the necessity for the extralegality of the emergency exception in times of crisis and peril (Gostin, 2003; Honig, 2009; Jennings, 2003; Lukes, 2006; Scarry, 2011).

The continuing viability of ordinary ethics during extraordinary times is a theme that is central to our notion of emergency preparedness as a civic practice. The ethical acceptability of an emergency plan is a function both of the substantive content of its provisions and of the process through which those provisions are discussed, formulated, argued about, and, ultimately, agreed to.

We would like to distinguish between two culturally available ways of understanding the content and the process of emergency preparedness. We call these the *civic perspective* and the *consumerist perspective*. We believe that emergency preparedness is best understood from a civic perspective, and it is this perspective that will inform our discussion of the ethics of emergency preparedness in this chapter. But it is important to grasp the difference between these two ways of understanding emergency preparedness, especially since the consumerist perspective is so often implicitly embraced when emergency preparedness is discussed and promoted, even within the public health field. Also, the consumerist perspective fits well with the background individualism and market orientation of American society today.

From a civic perspective, emergency preparedness planning and response are forms of activity that ordinary citizens ought to engage in out of a sense of membership and solidarity. Membership perceives that everyone is a part of a community of common interest and common vulnerability. Solidarity perceives that we have a responsibility for others and for the health of our shared community as a whole. From a consumerist perspective, emergency planning is fundamentally a specialized service that fearful and vulnerable individuals ought to purchase (as taxpayers) for their own protection. From a civic perspective, citizens engage in emergency planning and cooperate with its implementation. According to a consumerist perspective, individuals submit to plans devised and implemented by experts.

When viewed through the lens of the consumerist model, emergency planning is rather like medical or financial planning. Providers with specialized knowledge are preparing a product for clients who are consuming (using) that product to promote their own interests as consumers. When seen as a civic practice, on the other hand, emergency preparedness is not a commodity to be exchanged between a consumer with an interest and a provider with the expertise to fulfill that interest. It is part of the public function of protecting and promoting the security, life, liberty, and well-being of the people as a whole (Benjamin, 2006; Schafer, Carroll, Haynes, & Abrams, 2008). An emergency plan is not the property of those who create it; it is not simply "used" by the people who benefit from it. It is an expression of the entire community about the value of the lives and health of its members. It is less like a contract between seller and buyer (provider and client) and more like a covenant, an agreement to be entered into by all and that establishes commitments of responsibility for each (Vawter et al., 2010*a*; Vawter, Garrett, Gervais, Prehn, & DeBruin, 2010*b*).

If emergency planning is viewed as a civic practice, then citizens are parties to the plan, not consumers of it. Hence, from the civic point of view, it is entirely appropriate to emphasize broad, inclusive participation and community engagement in the planning process. Emergency preparedness is one important aspect of the life of strong democratic communities (Garrett, Vawter, Prehn, DeBruin, & Gervais, 2009; Garret et al., 2011).

Some caveats are in order at this point. In stressing civic considerations in this conception of emergency preparedness, we do not mean to suggest that emergency planning should wait until preexisting barriers to full inclusion, participation, and community involvement are overcome, or until the conditions of social justice and equality that make civic participation fully meaningful are achieved, or until broader social problems, like racism and poverty, are solved. Planning must cope with society as it is, not as it could or should be. And we do not mean to suggest that emergency preparedness will be the sole—or even the principal—instrument of social reform. Many other activities must converge on the problem of civic renewal and resilience. Nonetheless, we do believe that emergency planning can reinforce our civic life and our liberal democratic values (Childress & Bernheim, 2003; Jennings, 2007*a*, 2007*b*; Zack, 2009). To do so, it needs to be structured and carried out in a participatory fashion and not merely in the service of narrow health and safety goals, which the consumerist model highlights.

Civic renewal is a practical task, and people will not become involved in their community unless they find the activities and issues meaningful in their own lives and believe that their involvement will actually make a difference. Still, danger focuses attention, and public health matters—from bioterrorism to pandemic influenza to *E. coli* contamination—are coming to the forefront of public awareness. Because we are going to engage in massive and expensive efforts to develop emergency response plans in communities throughout the country, plans that will merge with climate change adaptation, why not get as much civic benefit out of the activity as possible?

Emergency preparedness is not only about protecting a community; it is also ultimately about embodying both the remembered traditions and values of a community and a forward-looking vision of how the community can be made a better environment for all its members in the future. At its best, emergency preparedness preserves the past, protects the present, and promotes a more secure, resilient future. Successful emergency planning must tap a preexisting fund of civic responsibility, a sense of justice, and concern for others in need. But emergency planning does not simply presuppose these virtues, it can—and should—be an occasion to foster them, as well. Fear and self-interest will no doubt be strongly in evidence during any public health emergency. But public health leadership can move communities beyond these motivations to a sense of common purpose and solidarity.[2]

Compass Points for Emergency Preparedness as Civic Practice

Emergency preparedness in each of its phases—the pre-event planning phase, the response phase, and the recovery phase—is a complex ethical undertaking, just as it is a complex managerial and scientific one. Ethical analysis cannot reduce that ethical complexity, and it does not pretend to offer a decision-making or policy-making algorithm. However, it does provide conceptual tools for discussion and clarification leading to agreement and common resolve. In that sense, ethical analysis may serve to enhance our capacity to prepare for and respond to emergencies in just, responsible, and effective ways.

The seven ethical goals discussed in this section are based on the notion that the emergency preparedness process ought to be guided by explicit ethical values that are commonly accessible and reasonable, albeit subject to ongoing interpretation, clarification, and discussion. As previously mentioned, these goals are not intended as rules or principles that must be followed in order to arrive at ethically correct decisions. That is not their purpose. But these goals do provide an orientation to guide emergency preparedness policies and activities. They are the compass points, so to speak, of a general orientation and mode of thinking designed to increase the likelihood that public health emergency preparedness will be both effective and trustworthy. This orientation is a civic one, and, when informed by that orientation, public health emergency preparedness can aim both to achieve ethically appropriate ends and to do so using ethically appropriate means.

The ethical goals of emergency preparedness are multiple, difficult to prioritize, and may give rise to practical ethical dilemmas when they conflict. (The same is true of ethics in virtually any area of practice.) They must be clearly articulated and understood for several reasons. These goals are intrinsically important, they express the values of the profession of public health professional service and traditions, and they represent the nature of a community's moral ideals. The clarification of these ethical goals is also important because widespread public recognition of them reinforces public trust and the legitimacy of emergency preparedness:

- *Harm reduction and benefit promotion.* Emergency preparedness activities should protect public safety, health, and well-being. They should minimize the extent of death, injury, disease, disability, and suffering during and after an emergency.
- *Equal liberty and human rights.* Emergency preparedness activities should be designed so as to respect the equal liberty, autonomy, and dignity of all persons.
- *Distributive justice.* Emergency preparedness activities should be conducted so as to ensure that the benefits and burdens imposed on the population by the emergency, and by the need to cope with its effects, are shared equitably and fairly.
- *Public transparency and inclusiveness.* Emergency preparedness activities should be based on and incorporate decision-making processes that are inclusive, transparent, and accountable so as to sustain public trust.
- *Community resilience and empowerment.* Emergency preparedness should develop resilient as well as safe communities. Emergency preparedness activities should strive toward the long-term goal of developing community resources that will make them more hazard-resistant and

allow them to recover appropriately and effectively after emergencies.[3]

- *Public health professionalism*. Emergency preparedness activities should recognize the special obligations of certain public health professionals and promote the competency of these professionals and coordination among them.
- *Responsible citizenship and civic commitment*. Emergency preparedness activities should promote a sense of personal responsibility and citizenship.

Saving Lives and Preventing Harm: A Broad Mandate

Emergency preparedness activities should protect public safety, health, and well-being. They should minimize the extent of death, injury, disease, and suffering during and after an emergency. It is important to notice the difference between the public health perspective on this objective and the perspective traditionally adopted by clinical medicine. What has been termed the "rule of rescue" is very powerful in social and medical morality. Saving lives has a very high—sometimes the highest—priority. "Above all, do no harm" (*primum non nocere*) is also an enduring tenet of medical ethics. However, the public health ethical objective of emergency preparedness does not focus solely on efforts to minimize the morbidity and mortality of isolated individuals; it must also protect the health of the larger population and community and promote the common good of all. Accordingly, the objective of minimizing mortality may sometimes have to be subordinated to other objectives. Faced with a pandemic, infection control may take precedence over the treatment of those already ill and at high risk of death (Battin et al., 2009). This will have a direct bearing on how vaccines and life-sustaining treatment (ventilators, or intensive care units) are used (Altevogt, Stroud, Nadig, & Hougan, 2010; DeBruin et al., 2010; New York State Workgroup on Ventilator Allocation in an Influenza Pandemic, 2007; Vawter et al., 2007, 2010*a*; Vawter, Garrett, Gervais, Prehn, & DeBruin, 2011).

Minimizing psychological harm and trauma is equally important. In addition, public health emergency planning must be concerned with minimizing economic loss, destruction of property, and the disruption of basic social services. Emergency preparedness should be conceived and practiced in such a way that it casts a very broad net. The importance of this has been demonstrated repeatedly (Jensen, 1997; United Nations, 2004).

Moreover, the scope of emergency planning does not stop there. It includes environmental damage, loss of biodiversity, and ecosystemic degradation. Such matters have both short- and long-term effects on public health (Center for Health and Global Environment, 2005; Frickel, 2006; Frumkin & McMichael, 2008; Sze, 2006). Consider some examples. As devastating as the injury and loss of life were on that day, they were not the only public health disaster on September 11, 2001. The other, ongoing disaster was environmental: the effects of the collapse of the massive twin towers and the subsequent human exposure to toxic materials during the event and for months thereafter (Langewiesche, 2002; World Trade Center Health Panel, 2007). Similarly, it was not so much Hurricane Katrina itself as it was the collapse of the levies and the resulting flooding that brought New Orleans into a public health crisis. And even that was exacerbated by underlying social, economic, and cultural conditions (Daniels, Kettl, & Kunreuther, 2006; Gilman, 2006; Graham, 2006; Hartman & Squires, 2006; Molotch, 2006; Strolovich, Warren, & Frymer, 2006; Tracy, 2007).

Thus, emergency preparedness must include not only planning for a catastrophic event per se, but it also must include upstream assessment and preventive measures and downstream recovery and mitigation. Building codes and their enforcement, as well as the proper maintenance of the aging infrastructure of US cities, are also components of emergency preparedness for they, too, protect lives and defend health. The connection between these upstream environmental and infrastructure issues and public health should be explicitly recognized and acknowledged because their importance is often forgotten, and other factors like cost savings and political expediency often overshadow them (Frumkin, Frank & Jackson, 2004).

Finally, the goal of harm reduction must be broad enough to encompass the social and cultural dimensions of catastrophic events and how they are planned for and responded to in both the immediate event and in the long term (Hoffman & Oliver-Smith, 2002). Emergency preparedness should strive to minimize long-term loss of social capital, cultural disintegration, and social suffering. Both the bio-psychosocial model of health that is widely accepted within the public health field and a growing body of epidemiologic research indicate that the destruction of webs of supporting relationships and of civic institutions can have significant effects on population health and well-being. All-hazard emergency planning and response must protect not only the whole person (i.e., both body and mind), but also organizations, systems of social functioning, and culturally meaningful ways of life.

An emergency plan is not simply a document: it is a process and activity itself, stretching over several years and revisited periodically. Plans should not only be reviewed at regular intervals for currency, but they should also be evaluated using exercises or drills. Emergency planning sets in motion a whole social complex—discussions, large meetings, small meetings, networks among officials and professionals, local organizing and educational activity, creation of new communication channels, and recruitment of specialized personnel or retraining of existing personnel.

The paradigm of emergency preparedness that provides the most latitude for achieving high ethical standards and ideals is a broad social model of emergency planning. It brings public health into contact with similarly oriented perspectives and movements in cognate fields. It draws orientation from social epidemiology and "place-based" (ecosystem landscape and built environment) public health, community-based participatory research, deliberative planning, and the building of learning communities and learning organizations in management and leadership science (Berkman & Kawachi, 2000; Forester, 1999; Schön & Rein, 1997). It may even have an analog in law enforcement and criminal justice theories of community policing (Friedmann & Cannon, 2007).

This is a broad mandate and a daunting task for emergency preparedness. Nonetheless, from an ethical as well as from a public health point of view, nothing less than this broad mandate and mission for planners will be truly adequate.

Respecting Individual Liberty: The Challenge for Emergency Preparedness

The noted political philosopher Sir Isaiah Berlin captured the core of the modern understanding of liberty as personal autonomy and self-determination when he wrote: "The defense of liberty consists in the 'negative' goal of warding off interference" (Berlin, 1969, p. 127).[4] In an emergency, it becomes difficult for an individual to be at liberty in this sense because being interfered with by someone or something is virtually unavoidable. It becomes difficult for each individual to respect the similar liberty of others, to leave them alone, or to stay out of their way. In an infectious disease emergency, each person becomes a potential or actual "vector" of disease transmission (Battin et al., 2009). In a mass casualty event, each person in need of medical treatment becomes an interfering or competing presence from the point of view of others who are injured and in need of special attention also. In an evacuation event, each car on the highway becomes an obstacle to the safe escape of others.

There is a long tradition of civil liberties in the United States and in many other countries, but ethics and the law have always recognized that rights and liberties can be temporarily overridden during an emergency situation when substantial harm to others is impending. Such temporary power has the potential for being extended in unjust ways and abused. A sensitivity to past abuses within public health itself has grown, and public health planners are—or should be—acutely aware of past restrictive measures that were justified on grounds of public health necessity but were later revealed to be instances of outright racism, social animosity, and invidious discrimination (Bayer & Fairchild, 2004). "Necessity" can be a value-judgment rather than an objective fact. Moreover, authoritative claims about necessity, especially in a crisis situation, can be used to shut down deliberation and lead to premature closure in considering policy options. It is an ethical mistake to be underinclusive in imposing restrictive measures because excess harm may result, but it is also ethically wrong to be overinclusive, for then the important values of liberty and rights have been sacrificed to no purpose of corresponding moral weight.

In 2001–02, these difficult issues were brought out in the open and made the subject of a wide-ranging debate by a joint project between the Centers for Disease Control and Prevention (CDC) and a team of legal scholars from Johns Hopkins University. This project produced the Model State Emergency Health Powers Act (Center for Law and Public's Health, 2001). A review of existing state laws found much inconsistency and many instances in which state authorities might not have a legal basis for taking the steps required in a public health emergency. The Model Act identified a wide range of powers to be granted to state governors, for a limited time, in the event of a properly declared emergency. Involuntary quarantine, invasive medical treatment without patient consent, the commandeering and destruction of private property by the state—all of these legally extraordinary practices and more were proposed for debate.

One of the principal authors of the Model Act argued that its measures are in keeping with a long-standing legal and ethical framework in the liberal democratic tradition in which personal liberty is balanced against preventing harm to others, and the interests of particular individuals are balanced against the public interest (Gostin, 2003; Gostin et al., 2002). Central to this analysis is the notion of a threshold restriction on individual liberty. Policy and public health authority should calibrate the lowest threshold of restriction that is compatible with meeting the public health and safety objective in question.

Similar notions are in fact widespread in public health ethics and in ethics generally. The maxim of utilizing the "least restrictive alternative" or the "ladder of intervention" is a way of simultaneously minimizing harm and respecting freedom in an emergency (Holland, 2007; Nuffield Council on Bioethics, 2007; Upshur, 2002). However, this idea is limited by the fact that it seems to presuppose that it is known where the objective threshold of liberty restriction lies—for instance, what subset of persons to quarantine because they pose the true risk of spreading disease when it is not necessary to quarantine the entire group (Campion, 1999; Parmet, 2007).

Overinclusive restriction of liberty is problematic, of course, because it has untoward side effects (Annas, 2002; Fairchild, Colgrove, & Jones, 2006). It wastes scarce resources to maintain a large restricted population and to ensure compliance. It takes persons who have been unnecessarily restricted away from more productive activities. The core of the problem raised by the use of liberty-limiting emergency interventions, however, is that they override something that arguably is of intrinsic value and something that we all have a duty to respect: the value of individual liberty and the right of adults to make judgments for themselves concerning precautions, prudence, and balancing safety and risk reduction against other personal values and priorities (Annas et al., 2008).

It is tempting to say that when protecting life and respecting liberty conflict, one must err on the side of life. Public health professionals may feel that the protection of health justifies the restriction of liberty as well. Restrictions of liberty are most readily justified when the restrictions last only a short time, and the damage done to the person thereby is reparable or compensable. Material interests, such as confiscated or destroyed property or lost wages due to mandatory social distancing measures, are compensable; loss of dignity, failure to be treated as an equal and with respect, or suffering stigmatization and loss of privacy might not be. It is always important for those in authority—and this applies as well to those with benevolent motives—to recognize the fallibility of their judgment and the limitations of their ability to foresee all the consequences of public health policies that restrict individual self-direction and freedom of choice. The balance between preventing harm and respecting liberty is not as easily struck as it may first appear, particularly in the planning phase of emergency preparedness.

In addition to the idea of using the least restrictive alternative as a means to achieve a public health objective, borrowing the judicial notion of due process can be a guide for striking the right ethical balance under conditions of uncertainty. Emergency preparedness should respect the right of persons not to be denied liberty or property in an arbitrary, discriminatory, or unnecessarily restrictive way. The reasons for the restriction of liberty matter ethically. The infringement on liberty will not be as severe if the person being restricted perceives that the restriction has been determined in a fair and reasonable way. Many times, it is not the restriction of freedom of movement or freedom of choice per se that is offensive, but the suspicion that it represents a discounting of the worth of the person being restricted.

Similarly, not only the reasons why liberty is being limited, but the manner or way in which it is limited matters. Emergency plans and procedures should respect the privacy and confidentiality of individuals who have to be restricted and should protect them from undue social stigma and humiliation. Also, the balancing of liberty against other values so that respect for persons is not undermined can be achieved when plans make special accommodation and provision for those with special needs or impairments. Those persons will suffer disproportionate burdens or be denied rightful benefits if their impairments are not compensated for by environmental mitigations, special equipment, resources, or services.

Voluntary Versus Mandatory Compliance Policies

The issue of voluntary versus mandatory compliance policies has a specific bearing on the problem of ethically justified limitations on liberty. Emergency plans are replete with features that essentially tell individuals what they are expected to do under specific circumstances. In emergency situations, the stakes are high, and noncompliance has serious and sometimes immediate consequences.

For the most part, a voluntary compliance approach is ethically superior to mandatory compliance, assuming that the necessary behaviors can be achieved. For instance, self-imposed quarantine in one's home is ethically preferable to mandatory incarceration in a supervised facility. An approach that mitigates harm and risk can rechannel liberty without unduly restraining it. Social distancing orders without too much in the way of surveillance and enforcement is another example of an emergency procedure that treads lightly on personal liberty. Voluntary compliance has a strong role in public health emergencies because people are fearful for their own lives and health and see that the restrictions are beneficial; people also feel conscientiously the importance of not putting others at risk by failure to comply with the emergency plans requirements.

Nonetheless, when it is clear that individuals pose a serious risk to others by their unwillingness to comply with behavioral restrictions, there is clear ethical justification for compelling them to do so. Similarly, when there is reason to believe, on the basis of sound evidence, that large numbers of people in the population are unlikely to comply with various restrictions voluntarily (a curfew or home quarantine, for example), mandatory policies backed up by law enforcement are justified, although they should be used with the utmost restraint and judiciousness. Mechanisms for timely individual hardship appeals should be readily available.

Situations of justifiable coercion exist, but they should be arrived at gradually. Attempts at correcting misinformation and at rational persuasion should be made before more punitive or physical measures are used. This standard applies both in cases of harm to others, where ethical justification is relatively straightforward, and in the more difficult cases of noncompliance involving only harm to self (Conly, 2013; Gaylin & Jennings, 2003; Trotter, 2007).

In the emergency preparedness context, it is unlikely that too much time or energy will be expended on those whose behavioral limitations (or noncompliant behavior) pose only a risk to themselves. Rescue workers during a flood will not linger too long to persuade a person to leave his or her home when there are still many other people up the street awaiting rescue. Also, the scarcity of time and human resources raises the question of whether it is fair to others to take the additional time necessary to gradually work through the steps along the spectrum from persuasion to coercion. Moreover, attempts to use physical coercion by those not properly trained in such techniques will put both themselves and the noncompliant individual at risk.

If mandatory restrictions on liberty are ever chosen by emergency planners and policy-makers, they have a responsibility to ensure that adequate resources are available to enforce those requirements fairly and humanely. This is but one example of the general proposition that a part of ethically responsible emergency preparedness is to provide adequate training and materials to public health workers and other public safety officials and first-responders so that they can do their jobs effectively and safely. Risk inherent in the situation does have to be accepted by those who volunteer to serve, but risks that are artifacts of poor planning and policy are unjust and should not be imposed on anyone. One can easily realize how much emergency preparedness involves matters of ethics by remembering the consequences of not doing it well (Bytheway, 2006; Fussell, 2006; Oliver-Smith, 2006; Scanlon, 2006).

Justice and the Allocation of Resources

Perhaps the most pressing, difficult, and anxiety-provoking ethical issues prompted by emergency preparedness concern the problem of distributive justice. If a pandemic of avian influenza were to strike the United States, who should be given priority in the distribution of scarce vaccines, antiviral medications, and ventilators? When the next devastating hurricane overwhelms coastal communities, which affected neighborhoods or population groups should be evacuated first? Should society invest significant resources to try to rescue those who have chosen to remain in place? If the United

States experiences another anthrax attack, should antibiotics first be given to politicians or postal workers? In the face of death and scarcity of resources, the old questions remain as relevant and disturbing as ever: Who shall live when not all can live? How shall we choose who lives and who dies?

In addition to these urgent questions posed at the point of distribution in the trenches, society faces equally difficult policy choices concerning how much to spend on the production and stockpiling of medicines and materials in anticipation of a crisis, particularly when those resources will go to waste if a crisis does not occur as feared. Suppose policy-makers take the seemingly prudent course and decide to stockpile vaccines, antiviral drugs, antibiotics, ventilators, hospital beds, and other life-sustaining resources. How large a stockpile should they create, and at what cost? As the richest nation on earth, perhaps we should attempt to create a cache of goods so massive that it might preclude the necessity of rationing should disaster strike (Institute of Medicine, 2008).

However, given the equally massive opportunity costs involved in such an undertaking, the low likelihood of emergencies actually striking at any particular place and time, and the need to constantly replenish aging stockpiles of dated drugs, perhaps it would be better to de-emphasize the importance of stockpiling in favor of building up a basic public health infrastructure and hospital overflow capacity.[5] If it is decided to stockpile, how much of current public health and national budgets should be devoted to this enterprise, and what sorts of items constitute the best candidates for this purpose?[6]

Questions of justice often achieve special saliency in the course of emergencies because emergencies often feed upon and exacerbate deep-seated, chronic, and pervasive patterns of social injustice that precede them. Hurricane Katrina provided one of the most graphic illustrations of this phenomenon. Although that natural disaster wreaked havoc upon rich and poor alike, the poor and marginalized, neglected for so long, bore the brunt of the catastrophe (Cooper & Block, 2006). The faces of the displaced and desperate survivors in the New Orleans Superdome were by and large the faces of poor and middle-class African Americans who lacked the money or the means to escape from the rising waters. Many of the medically and socially worst-off citizens of that city, those with physical and mental disabilities and their families, never even made it to the Superdome, victims of drowning in their own homes or on the lower floors of abandoned facilities. Emergencies thus tend to highlight and exacerbate the deep social fissures and chronic social injustices that haunt our society.

Why Deliberating About Justice During Emergencies Is So Difficult

Even under the best of conditions, thinking about the nature and demands of justice is difficult and contentious. As with the value of liberty, fundamental questions of justice generate conflicting answers and rival "-isms"—for example, utilitarianism, egalitarianism, libertarianism, and communitarianism. Even beyond the usual problems posed by the essentially contested nature of ethical argument, there is ample reason to worry that thinking about justice in the context of emergency preparedness will face particularly vexing obstacles.

First, some might argue that thinking about just responses to emergencies is pointless precisely because emergencies, by their very nature, tend to overwhelm a society's capacity for rational thought and planning. Large-scale emergencies engender large-scale social chaos. Reliable information is scarce, resources are quickly tapped out, front-line responders are stretched to the breaking point, and the desperately needy in ever greater numbers cry out in anguish for rescue. In the fog of chaos, one might argue, thinking about justice is a distracting waste of time; the best we can do is rely on ad hoc, seat-of-the-pants judgments and muddle through as best we can.

Although the chaotic aftermath of any given disaster is a context particularly ill-suited to measured deliberations bearing on distributive and procedural justice, this does not warrant emergency interventions guided exclusively by considerations of efficiency, the greatest good of the greatest number, or a kind of amoral realism in which might makes right. On the contrary, the ability to predict in advance the fog of chaos makes it all the more imperative to engage in deliberation—"thinking in an emergency," as one scholar put it—about just responses to emergencies well before they occur (Scarry, 2011).

A second, more significant difficulty is posed by a question at the very heart of disaster planning: What share of the health-related budget should be directed at future planning specifically for various kinds of emergencies, and what share should be devoted instead to the establishment and maintenance of a robust public health infrastructure capable of providing sturdy all-purpose defenses against a wide variety of both current and future threats (Rosner & Markovitz, 2006)? Should government spend the greater part of its preparedness budget on shoring up the capacity of biological and chemical laboratories, which are used every day, or should it also invest heavily in building laboratory capacity against future radiologic attacks that might never take place? The danger here is that planners might be seduced into irrational thinking by the prospect of a threat that poses potentially catastrophic losses but whose probability of occurring is actually quite low.[7] Obviously, this way of approaching problems by focusing narrowly on the worst possible scenario can often lead to counterproductive results.

Unfortunately, there is no clear-cut ethical solution to this problem. Rational prudence would dictate some form of social insurance against the prospect of catastrophic disasters, especially for a rich country like the United States. Once disaster strikes, the public will want to know whether its worst effects could have been foreseen, and, if they could have been foreseen, why they were not prevented. In retrospect, spending additional millions of dollars in 2000 on shoring up the levees protecting New Orleans would have been the obviously prudent choice. On the other hand, spending millions or billions annually to prevent potentially catastrophic events with an extremely low probability of occurring might turn out to be the public health equivalent of the Maginot Line.[8]

A third problem underscores the more general issue of uncertainty in disaster planning. The inability to make accurate predictions extends not simply to whether or not a particular sort of disaster is going to occur, but also to the magnitude of all impending threats and to the particular populations or age cohorts that might be most threatened by them. Planning for a pandemic of influenza implicates many such uncertainties. Before a pandemic emerges from its incubator, health officials will not know what specific virus to target with a specially crafted vaccine, what range of effects antiviral drugs will have against it, and which age or population groups will be most severely affected (Arras, 2006). The lesson to be drawn from the existence of such pervasive uncertainty is that whatever conclusions we reach about the justice of any proposed mitigation activities must be considered provisional and subject to revision over time as the disaster unfolds. Flexibility in response to changing conditions and evolving knowledge will be crucial to successful emergency planning and emergency response.

A fourth difficulty for thinking about the justice of disaster responses stems from the existence of conflicting values at stake in such situations. The task would be considerably easier if emergency response implicated only a single overarching value, such as saving as many lives as possible. In such a case, planners would simply have to identify the dominant value and then array resources so as to afford it maximal protection. But, as we noted earlier in the section on saving lives and preventing harm, there are numerous countervailing considerations that make a simple rule of rescue or a maximization of any one value—even lives saved—problematic. One of those considerations is the fact of scarcity that throws into stark relief several conflicting values that vie for our attention and resources, both in normal everyday life and especially during emergencies.

In the example of pandemic influenza, priority setting with regard to the deployment of scarce vaccines or antiviral drugs might well be directed at saving the most lives, but priority might also reasonably be given to preserving vital social and economic services and infrastructures, to safeguarding the young rather than the elderly, or the disabled rather than the able-bodied. Here, too, there is no reliable societal consensus regarding the proper weight that should be attributed to some conflicting values, and this will make it difficult, if not impossible, to resolve rationally many disagreements over the justice of emergency mitigation activities. Many such conflicts involve tradeoffs between the maximization of certain values (e.g., lives saved or quality-adjusted life years [QALYs] secured) and the equitable distribution of resources. That is, in many cases, securing the "best possible" results, however defined, might conflict with exhibiting the sort of concern demanded by justice for every group potentially affected by these decisions. Such conflicts between achieving maximal efficiency and the equitable treatment of all concerned go right to the heart of just emergency planning and emergency response.

Conceiving Justice as Efficiency and Equity

For most of its long history, the field of public health has defined itself and its guiding orientation in terms of a population perspective. Whereas the focus of clinical medicine tends to be the individual patient, public health has focused on the health of entire populations, and whereas medical ethics has in large measure been guided by individualistic and deontological (duty-based and rights-based) norms of fidelity to the interests of individual patients, public health has gravitated toward a largely consequentialist and social welfare-oriented or utilitarian ethic focusing on maximizing population health. Traditionally, the norms animating the enterprise of public health have tended to place the safeguarding of public health and safety above the concerns of individuals whose condition or behavior might threaten society's well-being. In many ways, this focus on the maximization of good consequences comes naturally to public health, as does a utilitarian conception of justice that holds that a pattern of distribution of benefits and burdens across a population is just (or ethically justified on grounds of justice) when that pattern maximizes aggregate net benefit or provides a greater aggregate net benefit than any other practical alternative. For utilitarians, the maximization of welfare is the very definition of justice (Goodin, 1995).

However, the traditional ethical orientation of the field of public health has not defined justice only in terms of maximizing aggregate net benefit; public health is also deeply committed to a view of justice that is concerned with the fairness and the impact on individuals of the way benefits and burdens are distributed in society, as well as the aggregate results of that distribution. This equity or fairness emphasis on the protection of basic needs and rights of all individuals and groups has no doubt accounted in large measure for public health's traditional focus on the poor and dispossessed within society.

It is certainly possible to achieve both equity and efficiency under certain circumstances. Given the historical and epidemiologic correlation between poverty and disease, it should not be surprising that public health has adopted a special concern for the health needs of the poor and marginalized sectors of society. Whether one is attempting to combat the HIV epidemic, drug-resistant tuberculosis, or the after-effects of a devastating hurricane, the surest route to achieving maximal health returns is to focus attention on the plight of the poor, whose living conditions create efficient transmission of infectious diseases and increase vulnerability to natural disaster. Efficiency and health maximization are not the only reasons for a special focus on the poor and socially vulnerable, but they are powerful reasons nonetheless.

Justice as Efficiency: What Is To Be Maximized?

Conceiving of justice as efficiency or the maximization of results prompts the question: Maximization of what? Different answers to this question will yield different policy recommendations, both in public health and in emergency planning. First, one might view utility or general welfare as the maximand, which would lead to adopting a straightforwardly utilitarian theory of public health justice. In this view, actions and policies should be governed by social value criteria that include but transcend a concern for health outcomes.

In the context of emergency intervention, such a theory of justice would give priority not only to front-line public health workers but also to key political decision-makers and to workers in industries critical to economic welfare. Pushed to a logical extreme, such a theory could countenance prioritizing young healthy workers for pandemic influenza vaccine on the grounds that the greatest economic cost exacted by an influenza pandemic would be attributable to massive loss of life in the healthy working population.

In general, utilitarian theories of such broad scope are not appropriate for decision-making, either within health policy or public health, where the target of justice should remain focused on health outcomes. This would still permit planners to prioritize front-line public health workers, vaccine manufacturers and transporters, and other personnel indispensable for maintaining vital infrastructures both in health care and public health. Still, focusing exclusively or primarily on health outcomes creates the task of determining which health outcomes are the most appropriate target for public health mitigation activities in time of crisis. Should the maximand be some sort of quantitative measure, such as quality-adjusted life years (QALYs) or disability-adjusted life years (DALYs)? According to these methodologies, people rate various states of health and well-being ranging from 0 (death) to 1 (perfect health). Then, an emergency response's likely effect on quality of life (e.g., moving a patient from 0.7 to 0.9) is multiplied by the effect's duration and, finally, by the number of people thus affected. The cost per QALY can then be computed by dividing the estimated total bill by the number of QALYs promised by a particular emergency response. Formulas like this are intended to focus spending on those procedures that promise the most health-related bang for the buck.

Although methods of this sort have proved useful in setting priorities in health policy and public health, they remain highly controversial, primarily because of their tendency to obscure or preclude tradeoffs between the maximization of health and other important values. Critics charge, for example, that QALY/DALY approaches tend to give short shrift to the elderly and the disabled on the grounds that money spent on them will not generate as many QALYs as care given to younger people or to those who can be returned quickly to normalcy. The worry, then, is that such approaches are inherently discriminatory toward those who are often regarded as the most vulnerable or needy (Saunders & Monet, 2007; Vawter et al., 2007, 2010*b*, 2011).

A third interpretation of the object to be maximized would simply target the number of lives saved with available resources, regardless of the number of QALYs those lives have to offer. This simple and clearly stated objective has intuitive appeal. It would give priority to those who are most at risk for death or serious morbidity and to whose cure or rescue has the highest chance of success. Those whose rescue or cure would require extraordinary expense or who most likely would not respond to treatment (e.g., elderly, immunocompromised nursing home residents) would not be favored. A distributive principle framed in terms of saving the most lives would also avoid some of the problems inherent in more utilitarian views. For example, unlike some applications of utilitarianism that strive for maximal economic or social benefit, it would not give priority to politically and economically favored sectors of the society and would thus be less likely to erode social trust among the population at large.

Although the "most lives saved" metric meshes nicely with the population-based approach of public health, and although it might provide reliable guidance in many contexts, it, too, is vulnerable to the criticism that it ignores or precludes other important values. Like the QALY method and all conceptions of justice as the maximization of some value or other, this approach can be faulted in some contexts for ignoring the fairness of its favored distributions (Brock, 2004). In addition to producing the greatest amount of overall welfare, the most QALYs per dollar, or the most lives saved, a theory of justice is also expected to "give everyone their due." For some alternative approaches to justice, this will mean giving priority to the worst off or the most vulnerable, or ensuring that everyone has a fair chance at benefiting from a given distribution, or that everyone's basic, human needs are satisfied—regardless of the impact of such prioritization on our ability to maximize anything. Such alternative approaches are referred to as "duty-based " or "non-consequentialist" theories of justice that focus on the rule of equity or fairness.

Justice as Equity: Fairness for All

According to the equity conception of justice, these equity concerns can function either as external checks and balances imposed on the field of public health conceived as a health maximizing enterprise, or they can be embraced within an alternative, more capacious conception of public health as an enterprise at the service of social justice. With either interpretation, the traditional public health focus on the poor and marginalized can best be explained not simply as part of a health maximizing strategy, although it is surely at least that, but rather by viewing priority for the poor and marginalized as a demand of social justice (Powers & Faden, 2006). In this view, those whose basic needs have not been met by society, those whose fundamental human capacities have been systematically stunted by unjust social institutions have the greatest claim on resources at the disposal of public health.

At the very least, justice as equity would mandate various checks on the achievement of greater population health at the expense of individual rights; for example, through the precipitous isolation of infectious but compliant individuals. At most, it would claim that a concern for human rights is an integral aspect of the mission of public health. In the context of emergency response, justice as equity might mandate priority for the poor, people living with disabilities, and the socially isolated. Moreover, a more controversial equity-based view might give priority to saving the young (e.g., in a context of pandemic influenza) before the elderly, not on the convenient ground of social utility, but rather because justice demands it. In this view, the elderly have already lived (most of) their lives; they have already played out their "fair innings" (Williams, 1997). Children and young adults, on the other hand, have yet to live out their allotted span of innings and thus have a greater claim to public health resources.

The equity perspective thus complicates the task of doing justice in the context of public health emergencies. Whether equity concerns are viewed as externally imposed checks on the achievement of public health goals, as the traditional view would have it, or as internally articulated priorities of public health, the maximization of good consequences will have to be weighed and balanced against countervailing values. This tension poses a fundamental problem for a theory of public health justice because there is no consensus, either within society at large or within the ranks of philosophers, on exactly how such conflicts of value should be resolved. Most of us believe that equity concerns should temper the achievement of maximal health-related results, at least to some extent, but there is reasonable disagreement in many cases on how far the scales should tip in the direction of priority for the poor, the disabled, the vulnerable, or the young. What costs in terms of overall population health outcomes is a society willing to pay to safeguard the basic interests of various vulnerable groups? Even if we could all agree that those who are worst off deserve some degree of priority, concentrating resources on the desperately sick might in some circumstances be terribly inefficient at saving the most lives (Daniels & Sabin, 2002).

Suppose, for the sake of argument, that vastly more people could be saved during an influenza pandemic by targeting vaccines at school-aged children who quite efficiently transmit infectious diseases to their families and, in turn, to the society at large. Would justice demand that priority be given instead to debilitated, immune-system–depleted, elderly nursing home patients who might plausibly be defined as the most vulnerable group? It is not at all clear that justice would demand such a dramatic tradeoff with efficiency, defined as the ability to save the most lives. At this point, theories of justice appear unable to resolve such reasonable disagreements. Certain ethical principles might be clearly wrong (e.g., "Let the free market decide who shall live") or unfair in application (e.g., a lottery), but many proposed tradeoffs between the maximization of health and conflicting equity concerns appear to fall within a range of ethical acceptability, even if none may strike us as uniquely just or ethically correct.

From Substance to Process

Because theories of justice do not yield univocal solutions to such balancing problems, political philosophers are increasingly recommending processes of democratic deliberation as a crucial supplement to substantive theory (Daniels & Sabin, 2002; Fleck, 2009; Gould, Biddle, Klipp, Hall, & Danis, 2005; Gutmann & Thompson, 1996). In this view, a number of possible tradeoffs might be plausibly justified by conflicting sets of values, so the task is to formulate fair rules for a process that will serve to legitimate a particular social choice. The focus here is not on theoretical correctness, although it is often assumed that all the live policy options on the table will be "just enough" or not demonstrably unjust; rather, the focus is on legitimacy, or the question of why free and equal citizens should accept any given political decision, especially those bearing on tragic choices of life against life. All persons believe that their life is of equal value to the lives of others, so if any particular tragic choice favors others over us or our loved ones—if a decision has been made to give a ventilator or vaccine to someone else and if we are likely to die or suffer greatly because of that choice—we will certainly insist on knowing who made the decision and what reasons have been given to justify it. Above all, we will seek reassurance that the decision was fair and that it was reached by a fair process.

Typical requirements for fair process include:

- *Publicity or transparency in decision-making.* Contrary to those who believe that such tragic choices will prove socially toxic to a public unwilling or unable to contemplate them (Calabresi & Bobbitt, 1978), the partisans of deliberative democracy hold that when it comes to matters of social justice, and especially to matters affecting who shall live and who shall die, publicity and transparency about the grounds for decisions is a prerequisite of their legitimacy. Those who might have to pay the ultimate price of rationing decisions have every right to know how those decisions were reached and on what grounds. Secrecy or the rule of experts behind closed doors is by nature an unaccountable decision procedure that can obscure all manner of stupidity and injustice, including favoritism for one's family or social group and discrimination against minorities or the socially marginalized. Thus, in addition to being a precondition of legitimacy, publicity can help guarantee that decisions will be as well-informed as possible and, hence, will tend to be more substantively correct or just over time than decisions reached in secret. As an example, an economic study has been unable to document a single instance of large-scale famine in open, democratic societies with a free press. By contrast, examples of famines or horribly managed natural disasters are depressingly easy to document among secretive military regimes (Sen, 1983).

- *An appeals process*. Those who disagree with a certain value ordering or who believe they or others have been unfairly disadvantaged by a social choice should be able to appeal the decision to responsible and responsive authorities. This will help ensure that principles are being fairly applied and that decision-makers remain open to the lessons of new experiences and arguments. The existence of an appeals process testifies to belief that all persons are equal in moral status and have a right to have their grievances aired and addressed. When conjoined to the publicity condition, the appeals requirement can provide society with a public record of criticisms bearing on allocation criteria and of official responses to them. (Obviously, an appeals process without a publicity condition would be useless because one would have no idea what exactly to protest.) This sort of record can function analogously to the body of appellate decisions in common law systems like that in the United States, where principles constantly undergo reinterpretation and specification in light of new fact patterns and fresh perspectives on value orderings. Public scrutiny of this public record of criticism and official response could help detect and rectify inconsistencies in past patterns of decision-making, and public officials would have to either abandon or defend such choices (e.g., on the grounds of differing circumstances). Ideally, the result could be a growing body of increasingly sophisticated, morally justified, and politically legitimate case judgments that could inform future policy.

- *The relevance condition*. Some defenders of deliberative democratic procedures have proposed that limits be placed on the kinds of reasons that might legitimately be advanced in such public deliberations (Daniels & Sabin, 2002). The only reasons that should count in public allocation decisions in health care or public health are those that could be accepted as relevant by fair-minded people who are disposed to find mutually justifiable terms of cooperation. Perhaps more sharply put, this means that appeals to reasons, evidence, or principles that could only be accepted by those already committed to some sectarian (i.e., religious) viewpoint will be ruled out of order.

This limitation on public deliberation is suggested for two reasons. First, coming to broadly acceptable social decisions on such morally and politically fraught issues is difficult enough without having to wade through fundamental and rationally irreconcilable religious commitments bearing on life, death, and our place in the universe. Second, the relevance condition is advanced in order to protect free and equal individuals from the imposition of public policies whose grounds (in sectarian religious doctrine) they could not freely accept. In the context of abortion and physician-assisted suicide, the imposition of sectarian religious beliefs upon the entire body politic has been said to amount to a kind of tyranny (Dworkin, 1993).

As opposed to the publicity and appeals conditions, this relevance condition is controversial and potentially problematic (Friedman, 2008). Although designed to simplify public deliberation by bracketing highly contentious religious appeals, this condition leaves in place many equally contentious claims emanating from ethical or political theory on which many reasonable people can and do vehemently disagree. As a result, the process of deliberation is not likely to be substantially facilitated by automatically discounting certain beliefs or arguments because of their religious provenance. In addition, many if not most, persons' approaches to questions of ethics and public policy are no doubt in large measure shaped by their own religious commitments. To officially rule out all such religious sources would thus have the effect of disenfranchising a large segment of the population from the deliberative process and would no doubt be interpreted by those excluded as a kind of demeaning marginalization. This problem could, however, be ameliorated somewhat by interpreting the relevance condition as excluding only those religious arguments that could not be given a secular translation. For example, religious arguments for racial integration and against legal segregation could be stated either in the language of the Hebrew prophets used by Martin Luther King or in the language of justice and equality. King's biblically based preaching for social and legal equality would thus not run afoul of the relevance condition.

- *Democratic participation and involvement of stakeholders.* A major theme in much commentary on democratic deliberation is the need for greater citizen participation in public policy decision-making. For policies to achieve genuine legitimacy in the eyes of the public, more is needed than publicity and an appeals process. Notwithstanding their crucial importance, those two conditions cannot do much to allay the perception on the part of many that life-and-death policies in emergency preparedness are unjustly or arbitrarily imposed from on high by distant bureaucrats or experts.

The primary remedy for this perception is greater involvement of the public in emergency preparedness policy formation. The guiding idea is that those whose interests are affected by public health policies, and especially those who are negatively affected, will be more inclined to view such policies as legitimate and fair if they (or others like them) have had a voice in the development of such policies. So it behooves decision-makers in government and public health to strive for enhanced public participation, not only because such participation is an intrinsic democratic value, but also because it is the best way to secure crucially important collaboration between public health officials and the public in a common, communal effort to secure the public's health in an emergency (see Chapter 4). The nonemergency context of the Oregon Medicaid reforms of the 1990s provide a good illustration of this point. Despite many warnings that the public could never accept transparent discussions bearing on the rationing of health care, Oregon seems to have been largely successful in its effort to solicit public engagement and support for explicit health care rationing (Bodenheimer, 1997; Fleck, 2009).

Although there is widespread agreement on the desirability of enhanced public participation in the policy formation process, there is disagreement on the exact form that such participation should take, who should be asked to participate, what should be the ground rules for discussion, what information should be provided, and how to judge the results. Moreover, merely inviting various stakeholders or community representatives to take part does not ensure that the requirements of democratic representation have been met or that the outcomes of the process are just. Great care must be taken to secure broad representation of affected populations, especially among those who are the least well off, the most in need, and the most marginalized.

Although we are not in a position to specify the details of how civic participation should be arranged and conducted in emergency preparedness, we view this as a crucially important condition for the legitimacy and acceptability of public health decision-making bearing on the allocation of scarce resources. We encourage emergency preparedness professionals to search for best-practice examples from communities that have faced disaster situations for guidance.

Justice Issues in Phases of Emergency Preparedness

Several different sorts of justice/allocation issues might arise during the planning, response, and recovery phases of emergency preparedness, and these will be briefly discussed here.

The planning phase is a crucially important period for integrating justice-based concerns into emergency preparedness. Because planners will not be able to deliberate in a serious or sustained way about justice in the thick of a disaster, they should be asking ahead of time what sorts of responses are ideally (or at least adequately) just and which processes for decision-making are ideally or adequately fair and legitimate. This is the period during which crucial decisions will have to be made about what sorts of resources and how many of each should be stockpiled for eventual distribution in a public health emergency. It is also a time to deliberate about the proper criteria for allocating scarce resources, to enlist the public's participation in this process, and to secure public support for whatever criteria are selected. This is the time for asking and grappling with the difficult questions, such as whether age should be a legitimate criterion for allocating ventilators or vaccines during a pandemic of influenza, and what percentage of the national wealth should be allocated to helping other nations cope with threats that implicate all countries, such as pandemic influenza. This process should take place at all levels in society, from town councils to state and federal governments.

If this job has been done adequately during the planning phase, substantive criteria for distribution and fair processes should already be in place awaiting deployment during the response phase. This is not to suggest that advance planning will obviate the need for thinking about justice in the thick of an emergency. Like war, public health emergencies have a way of foiling the best laid plans and wreaking havoc with carefully wrought protocols. Resources will be exhausted and personnel will be stretched to the breaking point, and no matter how much planning has taken place, health officials will no doubt be surprised and confounded by events at hand. Hard choices in the thick of disaster will have to be made.

In addition to the planning phase of emergency preparedness, the recovery phase is also a period when serious considerations of distributive justice, equity, and fairness should be factored into policy- and decision-making. Even as background social inequalities and special vulnerabilities may magnify the disruptive effects of a public health emergency on certain individuals or groups, so, too, will such background factors affect how readily certain segments of a community will be able to recover and rebuild following a disaster event or emergency situation.

Justice during the recovery phase involves allocation of scarce resources among individuals and groups in need, and it is closely tied to the notion of resilience at the level of entire communities. A community marked by just social practices and a commitment to social justice before an emergency is likely to carry that commitment through the emergency response and into the aftermath and recovery period. Such communities are likely to be better able to rebound quickly and recover effectively, and such communities will likely meet the benchmarks of both justice and resilience in their recovery process and outcomes. Resources will normally be scarce during the recovery phase, and the pace of rebuilding and recovery will not be the same for everyone who needs these resources and assistance. Priorities will have to be set concerning when and in what order people receive assistance, even if eventually there will be sufficient recovery resources to go around.

Policies and decisions that meet the ethical tests of justice will not place an undue burden on any one segment of the population in the recovery phase, and such policies will attempt to bring about as even-handed and uniform a pattern of assistance and recovery as possible. Generally speaking, priority in recovery efforts should be provided on the basis of greatest need and greatest impact. Those who will be otherwise homeless, for example, might be given priority on lists for temporary housing and shelters over those who have family or other private means of temporary housing assistance. Those at greatest health risk because of the dislocation of their ordinary routines and modes of living should be given special attention in preference to those who are experiencing inconvenience but are not being placed at serious risk. Those whose small businesses cannot survive a prolonged closure or period of inactivity might receive priority for available business recovery loans.

Not only the fact of recovery assistance per se, but also the nature and timing of that assistance are important factors in the distributive and priority-setting decisions in the response phase of emergency preparedness. An old saying in the criminal justice context, "Justice delayed is justice denied," can be adapted to a similar maxim for emergency preparedness: "Assistance delayed is assistance denied." This consideration bears especially on the mechanisms that are set up to handle the allocation and utilization of recovery assistance.

Here, considerations of justice cut two ways. On one hand, justice requires that waste, fraud, and abuse be prevented as much as possible so that assistance actually does arrive at its intended and appropriate destination. Procedural and administrative safeguards should not be lightly dismissed as mere "red tape"; they have an important ethical function in any public service setting. On the other hand, excessively restrictive, bureaucratic, and inflexible procedures during the response phase will also undermine the goal of justice. Health officials must not spend so much time determining whether a patient is eligible to receive a medicine that the patient deteriorates while waiting. They must not make it so onerous to restore business functioning, education, housing, environmental remediation, and other elements of recovery that a community expires from outmigration, capital flight, and social despair.

Meeting the Special Needs of Vulnerable Populations

Previous sections have focused on the ethical values of life, safety, health, liberty, and justice (as fairness and as welfare maximization) in the context of emergency preparedness. The theme that unites these various discussions is the reconciliation of respect for persons and individual dignity with service to the entire community and the common good. This theme can be deepened and explored more fully in the context of protection and service to those who, in an emergency event and its aftermath, will be especially vulnerable to harm and injustice—the loss of life, health, or dignity.

During a public health emergency, all persons experience unusual and often urgent needs for rescue, protection, vaccination, medical treatment, and other public health support. To that extent, any emergency makes everyone "vulnerable"; no one is completely self-reliant, and serious and urgent needs call for an ethical response of mutual aid, caring, and attention. Nonetheless, some persons and groups have background conditions and situations that compound their vulnerability during emergencies and expose them to special kinds and degrees of risk and disruption (Kailes, 2005*a*; Levine, 2004). These background conditions call ethically for special provision, accommodation, and concern.

The ethical goals of emergency preparedness understood as a civic practice all point in the same direction: persons and groups with physical, cognitive, or emotional vulnerabilities and those with social, cultural, and geographic vulnerability should be given special attention and recognition in the emergency preparedness process (Wizemann, Reeve, & Altevogt, 2013*b*). These individuals should not be left to "fend for themselves," even temporarily during an emergency. They may not be able to evacuate without special assistance; they may be particularly susceptible to infectious disease, which targets those whose immune systems are not only compromised by chronic illness or age but also by inadequate diet and other circumstances of poverty.

A concerted effort to anticipate and plan for addressing special needs and accommodating special vulnerabilities is an essential part of preparedness planning (Davis & Mincin, 2006; Drexel University Center for Health Equality, 2008). During the planning phase, this effort most often involves direct consultation with and participation of those with special knowledge or lived experience pertinent to individuals and groups who have such special needs. Then, during the response phase, an equitable use of resources and a genuine commitment not to abandon those at special risk must inform the decisions and mitigation activities during the emergency response phase and its aftermath. Finally, the concept of vulnerability and special need should continue to be taken into consideration and recognized during the recovery phase (see Chapter 3).

Emergency preparedness cannot be a substitute for a progressive effort to improve services for those who are vulnerable or who have been pushed to the margins of society—those on the receiving end of racial and ethnic discrimination, those in poverty, those living with chronic illness and disability, or those in need of long-term care. However, it can at least try to ensure that persons and groups with special needs are not forgotten or abandoned in times of crisis or emergency; that they, too, will be rescued, protected, and provided for; and that they, too, may hope to survive an emergency and emerge on the other side to resume lives of dignity and meaning. Emergency preparedness can also benefit from the strengths and assets present in the neighborhoods and communities where vulnerable persons live because these communities often have the local knowledge, trust, and outreach capabilities that are essential to effective emergency preparedness.

The Concept of Vulnerability

The concept of vulnerably refers to social, economic, and cultural inequities as well as to biological impairments. Vulnerability may be a function of the genotype, physiology, or personality of the individual. However, the full ethical implications of vulnerability become apparent only when it is understood in a social context. Vulnerability narrows the options and undermines the practical capabilities of individuals to flourish in times of normal activities and to take care of themselves in the face of danger or disruption (Vawter et al., 2011).

Disasters tend to highlight and exacerbate the deep social fissures and chronic social injustices that haunt a society. Shortcomings in emergency preparedness and response are often a function of preexisting inadequacies in the public health infrastructure and in other service systems. The devastation of New Orleans and other areas along the Gulf Coast in 2005 after Hurricane Katrina vividly demonstrated that some individuals and groups are much less able than others to protect themselves and to take advantage of public health and public safety systems, even when those systems are functional and accessible (which they sometimes are not) (Strolovitch, D., Warren, D., & Frymer, P. (2006). It also revealed the moral shame of discrimination and unfairness that can easily arise when resources are scarce and systems are under unaccustomed stress (Cooper & Block, 2006; Gilman, 2006; Strolovich et al., 2006).

Although difficult to define precisely or to enumerate exhaustively, various types of vulnerabilities and special needs exist that can inhibit or even paralyze effective or appropriate behavioral responses during emergencies. Emergency preparedness must plan for and make special deliberate efforts in advance to accommodate them (Kailes, 2005*b*). Again, vulnerability is not limited to states of special physical or emotional dependency on others, such as may characterize those with sensory or motor impairments, those with developmental or cognitive impairments, those with mental illness, children, or those who are frail and elderly. Vulnerability is also a function of social, cultural, racial, linguistic, and geographic disadvantage. Physically able-bodied and mentally capacitated persons may nonetheless be living in a condition of social vulnerability and precariousness. This form of vulnerability can be due to such factors as racial discrimination and stigma, poverty and lack of resources, lack of access to functioning and empowering social networks, or living in an area that has lack of access to services and resources or lack of access to transportation.

For these reasons, diverse types of special planning and accommodation are needed in emergency preparedness in order to meet the goals of justice, individual liberty and respect, and sustaining or rebuilding of resilient communities. Vulnerability does not necessarily mean helplessness. Vulnerable individuals and communities are often healthy and resilient, with many assets and resources, although those outside the community looking in often misjudge these factors. This fact was compellingly depicted in the 2012 film, *Beasts of the Southern Wild*, which told the story of people coping with the aftermath of the post-Katrina flooding near New Orleans.

Finally, vulnerability influences the ways in which people interpret the meaning of their experience and their overall life situation. Emergency preparedness activities need to be culturally, as well as physically and medically appropriate. They need to take into consideration the existing memories, sentiments, and prevailing attitudes of the persons or communities in question, each of whom will have experienced their particular "vulnerability" in a distinctive way that must be acknowledged and honored if trust and cooperation are to be established. Much of this depends on forging proper relationships, effective and trustworthy partnerships, and open, two-way lines of communication between emergency planning officials and distinct communities and neighborhoods during the planning process.

The question of how an emergency plan ought to account for and accommodate the special needs of vulnerable populations provides a kind of microcosm in which most of the ethical dimensions of emergency preparedness can be found. The cultural and social components of vulnerability have often been overlooked or discounted in the field of public health emergency planning (University of Florida, 1998; US Department of Homeland Security, 2005; US Department of Justice, 2006; National Council on Disability, 2008; National Organization on Disability, 2008). That should change—and is changing—because the cultural and social components of vulnerability are significant in their own right, both for affected communities of class or color and for persons with disabilities, for whom social vulnerability, perhaps as much or more than biological impairment, is a significant risk factor in their lives (Drexel University Center for Health Equality, 2008).

Anticipating and Addressing Special Needs

These vulnerabilities come from many different sources and situations, including chronic physical or psychiatric disease; physical, sensory, or motor impairments; cognitive or emotional impairments; developmental immaturity or disability; physical isolation; social isolation; poverty and lack of material resources; lack of support systems and other social resources (e.g., homelessness); fear of contact with authorities (e.g., the reluctance of undocumented aliens to call official attention to themselves); and strong emotional reactions, such as fear or a desire to maintain the status quo of normal life and everyday routine ("I will not leave my home!" "What is going to happen to my pet?")

Several groups in particular will warrant more complex accommodations. First, research has demonstrated that racial and ethnic minorities suffer disproportionately in the wake of emergencies. They are more likely not to be adequately prepared and to experience more injuries, diseases, and deaths. Public health emergency planning must address these racial and ethnic disparities in preparedness (Pastor et al., 2006).

Persons with some types of mental illness find it difficult to plan ahead, may be oblivious to warnings, and, in some cases, may be fearful or paranoid about participating in mass events such as evacuations. Additionally, some people with mental health concerns do not consider themselves ill, will not self-identify beforehand, and may resent being asked to participate because of the stigma associated with mental health problems. Some may refuse to evacuate and may place responders at risk when they are sent back into dangerous areas to provide rescue.

Likewise, persons with certain intellectual disabilities or other medical conditions that interfere or limit ordinary cognitive functioning may be particularly hard to reach (e.g., those with mild cognitive disabilities who may be living independently in the community). These individuals often are very isolated, have jobs with few friends or close colleagues, and often find comfort in a very steady routine. In such cases, they will be less apt to leave a home or disrupt a schedule they know well. They may be more likely to ignore warnings to leave the area and may be particularly fearful about evacuating because they are unable to figure out the complex set of instructions about where to go, whom to contact, and what to take with them (Elder et al., 2007). The more stressful and confusing the circumstances, the more likely some individuals are to retreat to their home or apartment and try to stay put until the stressful situation is over. These persons, in particular, will need special outreach long before an emergency occurs (James, Hawkins, & Rowel, 2007; US Department of Justice, 2006).

For example, consider the situation of a family trapped in their home by rapidly rising flood waters. In the family is a teenage boy with autism. When rescue personnel arrive, they find that a great deal of time and special communication skills are required to coax the boy into the waiting boat. The rest of the family will not leave without him. Is it feasible to deploy personnel with such skills, even if the location of families with autistic children is identified in advance as a part of the emergency plan? If many other families are waiting for assistance, is it justified to use coercion—physical restraints or medical sedation without informed consent—to remove this family more quickly? (Molotch, 2006).

To attempt to give a general answer to such an ethical dilemma is difficult and possibly misguided.[9] Difficult judgments will have to be made on the scene, taking very particular circumstances and assessments into account. Tragic choices cannot be entirely avoided in the response phase of an emergency. What can be strongly affirmed, however, is that appropriate advance planning and early identification of special needs can reduce the number of ethical dilemmas and tragic choices of this kind that will arise during an emergency response. The human cost and suffering caused by poor planning and lack of preparedness is the foundation for the ethical duty to plan and prepare well.

It is also important that emergency preparedness take into account the population of isolated persons in a given area. This includes persons who, for cultural, geographic, or social reasons, generally do not fall into any other category. Examples are persons who travel from one area to another seeking seasonal work, those who are homeless and living on the streets, those who are part of religious or cultural groups who specifically avoid contact with the outside world, and individuals and groups that historically have avoided interactions with government agencies. Another example of particular vulnerability that should be factored into emergency preparedness, especially during the planning and recovery phases, is illustrated by the impact of Gulf Coast hurricanes on the resident Vietnamese communities. Many in these communities are dependent on the fishing industry and have difficulty accessing services for linguistic reasons.

These and countless other examples are reminders that vulnerability takes many forms and manifests itself in many different ways. Personal health and safety may be put at risk; people may be displaced from their homes and supportive communities; people may be displaced from the broader economy; and people may, for linguistic or cultural reasons, be isolated from the mainstream sources of communication and social support services.

Those in charge during an emergency should have information concerning the number or location of isolated and otherwise vulnerable persons if preparedness planning has been done properly. But, during an emergency response, they must be able to retrieve that information quickly and act on it rapidly. Thus, it is crucial to keep such information up to date and maintain it in a form that will be accessible in an emergency.

This may require close and culturally appropriate cooperation with established ethnic, religious, and minority groups in the community, and such special outreach measures should be anticipated and planned. In many communities, for example, a kind of census of special circumstances and needs (e.g., housebound individuals) is taken by volunteers on the neighborhood level. This information is then communicated to public health and other government agencies, such as volunteer fire departments, so that they are better able to plan in advance to meet those special needs during an emergency.

In emergencies, when transportation is difficult and telecommunication unreliable, local emergency responders must have precise local knowledge concerning detailed special needs and precise physical locations. Links to such groups can be established beforehand by local emergency personnel, but, in times of emergency, proactive contact and outreach by authorities to these groups is essential. It cannot be assumed that they will receive information through media or through outreach by community-based groups, such as faith-based organizations, existing social networks, or volunteer groups.

Communicating emergency information to geographically and socially isolated individuals and groups may be especially difficult (Falkheimer & Heide, 2006). Some may avoid, or not have access to, mass media. Some may live in temporary quarters and not know the local area well enough to be able to follow evacuation information or instructions. Those who are isolated from others—for example, someone living in a motel at the edge of town for a couple of weeks or someone with a mental health problem living on the streets—may not interact with others on a daily basis or hear about a disaster or an upcoming emergency. Prior listing of where isolated individuals and groups exist in the community and advance identification of a specific person (perhaps with special training) assigned to follow up in times of emergency, may help reach out to these people. Those who work directly at the street level with isolated, displaced, or homeless persons probably have the most information and rapport with this population, and they can be a valuable resource for emergency preparedness planning.

Recommendations for Preparedness Planning for Vulnerable Populations

Persons and groups with special susceptibility to harm or injustice during public health emergencies exist in virtually every community and should be carefully identified and assessed during the planning process undertaken prior to emergency events. Without such pre-emergency event preparation, their special needs are unlikely to be met on an ad hoc basis during an emergency in progress. Advance planning and preparation are vital to protect these individuals:

- *Emergency preparedness planners should consider establishing a system whereby individuals with special needs and vulnerabilities can voluntarily register or otherwise identify themselves to local public health officials.* Alternate mechanisms are important because the formal process of registration may deter many people from participating. Enlisting the aid of well-trusted and respected community-based organizations is a key to emergency preparedness effectiveness. Such an approach begins with a general information and education effort to alert the community to the existence of the registry system and to answer their questions and concerns about it.

In most communities, there will probably then be two additional phases. The first will be an initial (and ongoing) voluntary phase during which individuals in the community take the initiative to put themselves into the registry. This should be accomplished in a variety of ways and made as convenient as possible. In the second phase, an effort is made to include those who do not voluntarily self-identify. One way to accomplish this is to enlist the cooperation of neighborhood and community groups, such as clinics; local physicians; senior centers; independent living centers; churches; trusted voluntary organizations in the community that offer special programs, shelters, and services; and local chapters of groups serving those with chronic diseases.

The creation of special-needs databases for planning purposes raises a number of ethical questions. Should these lists be voluntary, as we recommend, or mandatory? What incentives to register, if any, should be employed? Should individuals be permitted to designate themselves as in need of special assistance, or should some more objective basis for creating such databases be used? How can such lists be kept up to date? Who should have access to the database? How can databases be more effectively shared in a timely fashion? Should there be one central (i.e., regional or state) database? How should all of this be managed to balance privacy and emergency needs?

- *Public health officials should identify and work with community partners who have gained the trust of racial and ethnic minorities in order to identify at-risk persons.* This should be a critical element of emergency preparedness because racial and ethnic minorities might be less likely to accept a risk or warning message as credible without confirmation of the message from their trusted interpersonal networks (Spence, Lachlan, & Burke, 2007; Spence, Lachlan, & Griffin, 2007). Another barrier to emergency preparedness is that racial and ethnic minorities might distrust government officials and think that they are hostile, if not apathetic, to their well-being (Elder et al., 2007; Wray, Rivers, Whitworth, Jupka, & Clements, 2006). Following Hurricane Katrina, for instance, undocumented immigrants avoided recovery assistance because they feared deportation (Carter-Pokras, Zambrana, Mora, & Aaby, 2007). As part of the planning process, public health officials should work with churches, grassroots organizations, community-based organizations, and voluntary associations to develop culturally and linguistically appropriate strategies to identify at-risk individuals. For example, many African American churches maintain health ministries, and these may be a useful means to identify members of their churches who are at risk.

- *Auditing and mapping community assets (i.e., individuals with particular local knowledge or groups with special trust and loyalty in the community) should be an integral part of emergency preparedness.* To acknowledge that certain individuals, groups, neighborhoods, or communities are vulnerable to severe risk and disruption during a public health emergency is not to say that such communities are lacking in all assets or resources. On the contrary, vulnerable communities are not helpless. They simply need special advance planning and accommodations in order to help and sustain themselves. This reinforces the concept that emergency preparedness is and must be a civic practice actively involving all strata of civil society and not simply a centrally planned and top-down effort made on a service provision (consumerist) or public safety model.

An important element of auditing and mapping community assets is assessing the community's cultural diversity to make sure that preparedness efforts are conducted in a linguistically and culturally appropriate manner to ensure that all community members are included. A cultural assessment would answer such questions as what racial and ethnic groups make up the community, what languages they speak, what are their cultural perceptions of risk and emergency, what are their preferences for warning dissemination, and what are the trusted organizations and institutions.

Emergency plans should anticipate the need to provide linguistically, culturally, and functionally appropriate informational and educational resources for vulnerable or dependent individuals, their family members, and others who care for them about what to expect in times of emergency. This can be done both as part of general public education in times of emergency and through targeted education. It is perfectly ethical to say, "Mrs. Smith, you have a child who is ventilator-dependent and a wheelchair user. If you hear reports that the area will be evacuated in advance of the oncoming hurricane, please prepare to have your family ready to evacuate 24 hours before evacuation is expected to begin for the rest of the population." Having someone aware of this for several months or even years beforehand—and not at the last minute—would certainly be an ethically acceptable approach.

The provision of culturally and linguistically appropriate information is critical to overcoming language and information barriers. According to 2005 US census data, nearly one-third of Spanish-speaking residents spoke English "less than well." However, most warnings about Hurricane Katrina were provided in English only. Language barriers contributed to information delays about the path of the hurricane, delays in evacuations, and difficulties in understanding emergency messages (Messias & Lacy, 2007). Dissemination of preparedness information in languages that reflect a community's diversity is an essential ingredient for ethical planning and implementation of emergency preparedness. To better assist people with limited English proficiency, emergency planners might develop partnerships with medical interpreters and learn how to work effectively with them or even integrate them as part of the preparedness team.

- *Public health planners should not overgeneralize or base emergency preparedness on stereotypes or unexamined assumptions concerning those with special needs.* The pitfall of stereotyping or overgeneralization of beliefs and attitudes should be avoided in emergency preparedness for all vulnerable groups—those who experience social and cultural marginality as well as those living with disability. Differences of cultural and geographic origin matter to people. Broad categories, such as "Hispanic," "African American," and "Asian American" are of limited value for emergency preparedness. A much more fine-grained understanding of local community and individual perspectives, values, concerns, and differences is required in this type of planning. Persons with disability are often ill-served by stereotypes and broad categories of classification as well, being often viewed, for example, as isolated individuals or as belonging only to special groups cut off from the mainstream. However, many people with disability do not see themselves as part of a single group, and this is particularly true for those who are chronically ill or disabled later in life. Most people with disabilities have family members or significant others who are not disabled and will not want to be separated from them.

- *To facilitate good planning, individuals with special needs or their representatives should have an opportunity to participate actively and directly in the emergency preparedness process.* Emergency planning should draw on sources of local knowledge and familiarity with the everyday life and habits of various cultural groups and neighborhood communities. People with special needs are not simply a "problem" for emergency planning; they can be a valuable resource for it as well. To date, the means of communication in the planning process have not been as open or as inclusive as they should be. Better communication is needed to enable emergency planners to understand the special needs and concerns of vulnerable members of the community. This can in turn lead to more effective planning because they will be able to anticipate behavior and response to emergency situations (National Council on Disability, 2008; Spence, Lachlan, & Burke, 2007).

In particular, making appropriate and equitable provision for vulnerable individuals and groups in emergency plans requires input from those with direct experience and with insight into the perspectives of those living under conditions of vulnerability, marginality, or discrimination. Avoidable mistakes and miscues will occur if good and well-established lines of communication have not been formed between the disability community and public health officials. A motto of the American disability rights movement is, "Nothing About Us Without Us," and this could well be the aspiration of other vulnerable groups as well. It is an appropriate reminder and rule of thumb for emergency planning.

Identifying those with special vulnerabilities and needs and setting up special services and accommodations for them in advance of an emergency is critical so that they will not be the neglected or fall between the cracks (Drexel University Center for Health Equality, 2008; National Council on Disability, 2008). Once scarcities begin to emerge in an emergency situation and priorities begin to be set, vulnerable populations are likely to be lost in a general sea of trouble and need. When many needs are calling for attention, the voice of the vulnerable is most likely to be drowned out unless it has been heard in advance and special provisions have been made. Direct participation or consultation in the emergency planning process by those with special experience or expertise concerning vulnerable populations can prevent these deficiencies.

Emergencies that call for rapid, large-scale evacuation measures provide many examples of this potential shortcoming of preparedness plans. The events surrounding Hurricane Katrina showed that large numbers of people in low-income areas do not own cars and cannot be evacuated unless transportation is provided for them. Officials also discovered that emergency transportation arrangements that had been provided for in preexisting planning were not uniform but worked differently in different parts of the city. In addition, they learned that many other circumstances faced by low-income persons can complicate evacuation planning. Those who do not have access to banking services, for instance, often keep their valuables at home and are reluctant to leave their homes for that reason.

Individual family situations also complicate evacuation, and planning must aim toward keeping families together. Emergency shelters need to accept and accommodate pets, or their function will be undermined. Also, many persons with disabilities, those in wheelchairs for example, will refuse to be evacuated unless they are taken out with their families. Public health officials need to know in advance where persons with disabilities and other special needs are located and have appropriate transportation available to get them out of the area (accessible vans for example), and they must be willing to evacuate nondisabled family members at the same time. The challenges continue when persons using wheelchairs reach shelters, for whom mobility requires a reliable electric power source. Another example is that of persons with cognitive or developmental disabilities who often have very set routines and will refuse evacuation rather than disrupt that routine. They may fear, for example, that they will lose their jobs if they do not show up for work. A prior plan and prior discussion at work could alleviate this.

- *Public health measures, such as social distancing, designed to limit the spread of infectious disease pose special problems for those who rely on outside help.* Persons with disability and working mothers with young children are often dependent on caretakers or others who come in and out of their households on a daily basis to do specific tasks or help with specific chores. When attendants or child care workers are too sick to show up, or they are barred by their agencies from providing care because of fear of an infectious disease, the consequences can be very serious (Uscher-Pines, Duggan, Garoon, Karron, & Faden, 2007).

Family members and others who regularly check on someone with a disability may not heed warnings about not interacting with others. They must weigh the possibility of infection versus the concerns about the immediate needs of those for whom they care. Unless alternatives are put in place (such as some sort of visiting nurse service), these caretakers understandably may not heed warnings to stay away.

There is an important connection between foreseeing and accommodating special needs and circumstances in emergency preparedness planning and the type of behavioral response and compliance with the plan that an actual emergency event may elicit in the community. Response efficacy, promoting the general welfare, and adhering to the principles of justice are all involved in advance planning to meet the special needs of the vulnerable.

Making special provisions for vulnerable populations will also have an effect on the behavior of emergency responders and many able-bodied adults, so the overall success of emergency response plans is affected by the planning steps taken on behalf of the vulnerable. In emergency planning, as in many other areas of social policy, doing well requires doing good.

Communication and Participation in Emergency Preparedness

Two distinct but closely related facets of ethically sound emergency preparedness are "transparency" and "inclusiveness." Both involve the relationship between planners and public health professionals (as well as other leaders, opinion shapers, and elected officials) and the general public—the community and citizenry whom emergency preparedness exists to protect and to serve. Transparency has to do with external communication—moving information from the planning organization to persons outside that process. Inclusiveness concerns the internal conduct of the planning process. Transparency has to do with the content, style, and timing of public communications; inclusiveness with the active role of community members or representatives in the deliberations leading up to the plan itself.[10]

Provision for both transparency and inclusiveness must be made in emergency preparedness; both are vital to ethically sound, accountable, and practically effective preparedness and response. Ethical considerations push emergency preparedness toward transparent, respectful communication with community members because they have a right to truthful information and because they need that information so that they in turn can fulfill their civic and personal obligations during a public health emergency. Ethical considerations also push emergency preparedness toward formal and meaningful inclusion of ordinary citizens in the planning process and decision-making. There are both principled and practical reasons for this. Individuals have a right to deliberate about and influence decisions and policies that materially affect their own safety, health, and well-being. In addition, open, inclusive, deliberative planning will build the necessary foundation of legitimacy and public trust required by an emergency preparedness effort. Finally, inclusive participation will provide for feedback and self-correcting mechanisms that will improve the efficacy of preparedness measures (see Chapter 4).

Transparency and the Communication Spectrum

Emergency preparedness communication may be thought of as a spectrum of message transmissions. At one end is the direct conveying of information alone, without embellishment. That information may be about environmental conditions ("A level-four hurricane is expected to make landfall in 12 hours at location X") or about instructions or commands ("When the alarm sounds, proceed to the nearest underground shelter; do not bring your pets with you"). Further along the spectrum is communication that conveys information but also conveys judgment, explanation, and rationale. This type of communication admits uncertainty and probability; it attempts to persuade rather than simply to instruct ("Residents are advised to fill bathtubs with clean water and prepare for the possibility of widespread power outages"). These two types of communication are essentially one-way circuits, from leader to constituent, from authority to citizen.

However, good communication is more than simply providing factual information, and transparency requires more than simply telling people what has already been decided. Communication should involve a two-way form of exchange and provide the resources necessary for the public reasonably to reflect on and come to accept or reject proposed planning decisions. Communication about emergency planning—as distinct from emergency response—should be like (very good) political campaigning—the Lincoln–Douglas debates, for example—not like listening to the weather report. Thus, further along the spectrum of communication are two-way communication and feedback loops. The general public is enabled to comment on the top-down messages they have received and to ask questions about them.

Even further along the spectrum is the area of communication in planning that involves more active and direct grassroots participation, wherein lay persons have an opportunity not only to react but to participate in forming the plan from an early stage. Community forums permit discussion that is proactive rather than reactive, and these forums can produce ideas and information that may be factored directly into the ongoing planning process. This "community consultation" or "public engagement" can make a significant contribution to planning communication as well as to the planning process. Properly done, it can promote both transparency and inclusiveness. Community consultation makes for more intelligent planning before an emergency and better compliance with the provisions of a plan during and after an emergency (Keystone Center, 2007; Schoch-Spana, Franco, Nuzzo, & Usenza, 2007). In this role, it contributes to the discovery of factual information and the making of evaluative judgments.

The special area of risk communication requires additional consideration (Krimsky & Golding, 1992). Public health information prior to and during an emergency is often complex, hard to comprehend and assess, and often uncertain or probabilistic in nature (Silver, 2012; Sunstein, 2007). Under these circumstances, communication is especially difficult because the message sent and the message received may be quite different. Recognizing this problem, some in public health might argue for tight control of information and release of only minimal information during emergencies.

Another line of thought, which is growing in influence and which we believe is more desirable, is to have confidence in the ability of the public to handle information and to appreciate frank admissions of uncertainty on the part of public health officials. The public, far from losing trust in officials due to such openness and candor, responds well to it, while responding quite negatively to secrecy and deception when it learns about them after the fact.

The days of public health mitigation activities that are nonconsultative and paternalistic are mostly behind us. In recent years, public health practice has moved from the command pole of the communication spectrum toward the deliberative and participatory pole (Buchanan, 2000). Yet many conceptions of emergency preparedness are built around benevolent authoritarianism and paternalism, and they draw on models of public health communication that rest on more or less manipulative incentives and behavior modification approaches (Thaler & Sunstein, 2008). This remains a lively area of debate within public health as a whole. The notion that public health professionals direct the communities they serve toward better health is giving way to the notion that public health cooperates and collaborates with communities and individuals in a joint civic pursuit of improved health.

Inclusiveness: Civic Participation in Emergency Planning and Recovery

The benefits of inclusiveness and direct participation in the planning process, at least by representatives of grassroots groups and engaged individual citizens, can be substantial (Garrett et al., 2009). Such participation can alert the planning process to concerns, cultural perspectives, and other vital factors that professional planners may overlook (Schafer et al., 2008; Schoch-Spana et al., 2007). A sense of investment in emergency planning may lead to better community coordination and, ultimately, compliance later on. Deliberation does not inevitably lead to consensus, to be sure. But it can broaden horizons and encourage a civic, public-spirited attitude (Chambers, 2003; Gutmann & Thompson, 1996).

Well-managed participation and inclusiveness can have the same effect as timely, honest, and candid communications in promoting public trust and legitimacy and, hence, a greater willingness to cooperate during an emergency. Indeed, without these things, public trust is unlikely in today's society. Normal channels of interest group bargaining and lobbying no longer enjoy public confidence; they have been discredited by spin, misinformation, and financial influence. Nothing will make cooperation and the maintenance of order during an emergency more difficult than widespread mistrust and suspicion of leaders and authorities (Wray et al., 2006).

There is not a sharp line between community consultation or town hall meetings concerning emergency preparedness, on the one hand, and the inclusion of community representatives in the planning process, on the other. This distinction has to do with the numbers of participants involved, recruiting them, and their qualifications for the task at hand. It also has to do with the distinction between input that is advisory and input that has some more authoritative status. Community representatives are never given veto power over important decisions, but once they are accepted into the process, emergency planners must accommodate their wishes and needs to a great extent. Because these individuals will have access to information that is not generally publicly available, and because their roles and identities are known so they become points of attention by the media, they carry some influence. The political costs for elected officials of neglecting them or pushing measures through over their opposition can be substantial.

The personality and style of individual community representatives and the external pressures they are under will influence the roles they play in the planning process. They can generate conflict and be a disruptive presence for experts and staff, which could have the unintentional beneficial effect of forcing staff to broaden their agenda and their ways of thinking. However, they also may want to play a disruptive role in the process in order to reinforce their power and standing with their constituency.

The converse of this type of conflict in professional–lay relationships is generally referred to by political scientists as "cooptation" (Selznick, 1949/1984). Here, the community representative is led, usually by subtle psychological means, to identify more with the insider professionals than with the external constituency or community. Professional and bureaucratic interests seem to merge with community interests. The representative ceases to represent the grassroots in the sense of protecting their rights and giving them voice. Instead, the representative internalizes the same paternalist attitude toward the public that many insiders have.

Neither conflict over hidden agendas nor cooptation is what the ethical values of inclusiveness require. These considerations point to the importance of the selection process for community representatives. In general, we support inclusiveness and lay participation in emergency preparedness. However, it is rarely desirable to politicize the planning process. Appointing community activists with their own independent agendas, therefore, is less desirable than appointing more independent, detached individuals who are respected and trusted by broad sectors of the community. Such persons are genuine civic leaders and are more likely to be guided by the common good of the whole community. They can contribute well to a planning process that is both effective and has ethical integrity.

Communication During the Response Phase

Thus far, we have considered communication and participation largely in the planning and recovery phases of public health emergencies. The response phase requires a different kind of analysis. For effective communication and transparency, the prime imperative is to provide the most reliable information available in a timely manner. During an emergency response, the conditions are not auspicious for deliberation and consultation. Fear, insecurity, and uncertainty about the immediate future are not conducive to thoughtful, deliberative participation by citizens in any case, and, during an emergency, panic may lead people to undervalue the rights and interests of minorities or those who are stigmatized. Blame, rumor, and stigma are normally rampant during a time of crisis, and emergency planners should anticipate and attempt to minimize these outcomes (Barnes, Novilla, Meacham, McIntyre, & Erickson, 2008).

Good communication during the response phase can dampen bigotry, counteract rumor, and prevent or minimize panic. It is important for public health responders to have a good working relationship with the local press and, in all communication, to resist the urge toward benevolent deception or withholding of accurate information. Transparency, candor, and openness will serve both ethical and practical objectives. Communication during the response phase has a direct bearing on the choices ordinary people make and the risks that they are subjected to. Emergency responders should recognize the potential consequences of their actions in this regard, and their ethical obligations are not set aside simply because they are working often under very trying circumstances. Good advance planning, clear lines of responsibility and communication worked out in advance, and a carefully built and earned reservoir of public trust will help. Absent this, it is unlikely that any response effort will go well. Even with these factors in place, response-phase communications will be replete with hard choices.

Transparency counsels emergency communicators to trust their audience even as they need the audience to trust them. The public does not expect infallibility from emergency preparedness; it does expect fidelity. Transparent emergency communications follow these rules of thumb:

- Acknowledge uncertainty.
- Provide follow-up information as quickly as possible.
- Advise patience and flexibility.
- Admit mistakes and move on.
- Provide advice that fits the context and can realistically be acted on.
- Do not abandon the community, and do not appear to be doing so.

Participation During the Response Phase: Volunteers

Community representation and grassroots participation mark inclusiveness during the planning and response phase of emergency preparedness. However, the major aspect of participation that arises in the response phase is volunteer participation in the implementation of response plans and in providing services and staffing. Volunteerism is a double-edged sword. On one side, it is one of the most admirable aspects of any emergency situation and, as such, should be encouraged and applauded. On the other side, it can cause managerial and technical nightmares and reinforce the adage that the road to hell is paved with good intentions.

Sometimes the sheer number of volunteers can overwhelm the beleaguered professionals at a disaster site. The safety of the volunteers becomes a new issue to reckon with. Planning should include the provision of resources to supervise, train, and use volunteers effectively. How essential their function is will vary from one emergency situation to the next, but to actively discourage or restrict them from doing something to help is highly undesirable from the long-term point of view of community well-being and morale, no matter how expedient it may be in the short term. We are reminded of the conflict that almost broke out between the New York City police and firefighters at the World Trade Center debris pile when the former had been instructed to prevent the latter from joining the search for buried victims (Langewiesche, 2002).

An interesting aspect of using volunteers during an emergency arises in the provision of medical care and in performing medical procedures. Many state laws restrict such activities to licensed physicians and nurses, but, with some relatively simple training, others may reasonably be permitted to perform medical tasks such as starting intravenous lines, performing tracheotomies, and setting broken bones. The performance of medics in the military during combat demonstrates that something less than a medical or nursing degree will suffice. However, statutory change will be necessary, and the training resources are not currently in place (Hanfling et al., 2012).

In addition, the question arises of altered standards of care and legal liability. If someone sustains a serious injury while being cared for in emergency settings that do not conform to the standard of practice of normal times, should they be able to recover damages? Will their ability to do so make it impossible to set up a volunteer program as a part of an emergency plan? Should limits be placed on tort liability to protect those providing care and services in good faith during special emergency circumstances?

Many elected officials, policy-makers, and public health officials believe that lawsuits, to say nothing of litigious attitudes, are out of place in the context of public health emergencies and other emergency situations. Many existing state laws contain provisions limiting liability and access to the courts, and other states are considering adding such restrictions. The Model State Emergency Health Powers Act contains such a provision, for example.[11] Yet the problem of responsible oversight and public accountability remains to be addressed. Officials should not be paralyzed by concerns about civil liability during emergency response, and volunteers should not be prevented from assisting by such concerns. However, what then would be the mechanism of quality control over the actions of volunteers and recent trainees? Tort liability is one such safeguard in the US system. Partly, this is a question of acceptable risk, and partly it is a question of a tradeoff between the ethical objective of reducing mortality and morbidity and the ethical objective of protecting individual liberty, autonomy, and respect for persons. Liberty (in this case, the right to judicial relief when one has been injured or wronged) and respect for persons are not to be set aside lightly, even when a person's life is at risk. If liberty is limited in the name of protection, then it is contingent upon society to provide protection and not cause injuries due to improper management.

No doubt new laws and regulations will be developed that will balance the need for new standards of care during emergencies and the need to protect victims from neglect and incompetent treatment. This problem is not limited to nonprofessional volunteers. During emergencies, even physicians might have to do things that they would never do, in ways that they would never do them under ordinary circumstances (Health Systems Research Inc., 2005; New York State Workgroup on Ventilator Allocation in an Influenza Pandemic, 2007). Further comment on the technical questions of how to achieve that balance in the law is not within the scope of this chapter. From an ethical point of view, although this remains controversial, we recommend that the balance be struck slightly in favor of limiting liability and encouraging the work of volunteers. Despite foreseeable individual injuries, this will be in the best interest of communities and of ethically sound emergency planning in the long run.

Does the Emergency Exception Preclude Transparency and Inclusiveness?

The legitimacy of public health officials is based on their objective qualifications and the objective outcomes they produce. Training and use of qualified staff are necessary but not sufficient conditions for legitimacy. Legitimate authority must also be accountable to the citizenry at large and to those most directly affected by decisions made by that authority.

Accountability also means transparency regarding the conduct of public health officials. Voluntary compliance with public health authority requires an understanding of the reasons and rationales for policies and a sense of trust that the public interest is motivating public health officials in their activities. These general considerations apply to public health at all times, but they are no less important in the context of emergency preparedness.

It is sometimes argued, however, that the time and resource constraints of an emergency situation make the ethical requirements of transparency and inclusiveness impractical or even undesirable. The notion of an emergency exception to the normal rule of law and governance takes an ethical form as what might be called the "emergency excuse" for using power in a style of benevolent authoritarianism and paternalism, for limiting liberty broadly, and for rejecting transparency and participation. This point of view excuses authorities for climbing the ladder of intervention very rapidly, two rungs at a time.[12] We hold, on the contrary, that the emergency excuse in fact has less traction in ethical analysis than many in public health believe. It does not provide good grounds for setting aside the kind of ethical objectives we have offered in this chapter for at least two reasons.

First, whatever validity it may have during the response phase of an emergency, it does not apply to the planning phase, when time constraints are not so stringent. The link between transparency and later compliance is an important consideration to bear in mind during emergency preparedness. Second, even during the emergency response phase, when decisions have to be made under conditions of imperfect information and rapid response is crucial, it is still ethically necessary to differentiate between the reasonable and justified exercise of authority and power and the arbitrary, improper exercise of authority and power. Time pressure should not be used as a general excuse or reason to give officials an ethical carte blanche; if it is, the emergency response effort will most likely lack coordination and become a power struggle that will undermine effective response efforts. Adherence to the ordinary rules of morality and to the ethical objectives set forth here remains essential in emergency situations, not in spite of the fact that time is short and emotions are running high, but precisely because of these things.

Professional Obligations

Health care workers and other health professionals play pivotal, front-line roles in emergency response, yet the risks and divided loyalties (to their patients and to their own families, for example) they sometimes face can create serious professional, personal, and ethical dilemmas for them. Anticipating the reaction of health professionals and first-responders to these strains is an important component of emergency preparedness. Emergency plans spell out duties for specific individuals and groups who occupy particular roles in the response process. They also rest on an implicit gamble that those duties, with a small number of exceptions, will be fulfilled. It is important to note that this gamble is usually successful. But lessons can be learned from situations in which assumptions built into planning turn out to be mistaken. Although the story of health care workers and SARS was largely one of remarkable heroism and solidarity in the face of a deadly epidemic, hundreds of physicians in China refused to return to their posts (Brookes, 2005; Knobler et al., 2004*b*). Many others around the world found themselves making anguished choices between serving the ill and protecting themselves and their own loved ones from the threat of deadly disease. Although SARS was eventually contained by rigorous infection control measures, including widespread quarantine, future public health emergencies, such as an epidemic of smallpox or avian influenza, could place health workers at much greater risk of severe morbidity and death. Beyond the level of individual practitioners, individual hospitals might shut their doors to new patients because of fears that they might contaminate existing patients.

Do health care providers have a moral obligation to risk illness and death in the line of duty, not merely in routine situations involving infectious disease, but also in the broader disruption of a major disaster or public health emergency? Do physicians, public health workers, nurses, and others have a moral duty to stay at their posts in the face of risk, or are such choices merely a matter of individual conscience for individual practitioners (Vawter, Garrett, Prehn, & Gervais, 2008)? One philosopher put the argument this way: "Society's granting of power and privilege to the professions is premised on their willingness and ability to contribute to the social well-being and to conduct their affairs in a manner consistent with broader social values" (Frankel, 1989). But if the conduct of professionals like physicians and nurses is governed by a special ethic of professional duty, how strenuous is this duty, and what are its limits?

Of course, such questions are not new. They were routinely faced by physicians and nurses before the advent of antibiotics, especially during times of plague and outbreaks of other infectious diseases. In 1912, the Code of the American Medical Association (AMA) stated that, during such times, "a physician must continue his labors for the alleviation of suffering people, without regard to the risk to his own health or to financial return" (Baker, Caplan, & Latham, 1999). This principled stand was greatly attenuated, however, both by the AMA's increasing emphasis on physicians' untrammeled discretion in deciding whom to serve and, even more importantly, by the advent of the era of antibiotics, which gave the appearance of having forever vanquished life-threatening infectious diseases. During the brief period between the widespread dissemination of antibiotics and the rise of AIDS, the notion of a strong professional duty to treat in the face of mortal threat no longer seemed relevant to the medical community. But, as AIDS, SARS, Ebola, and the disturbing threat of pandemic influenza have amply demonstrated, the *pax antibiotica* was only a momentary reprieve, and the age-old questions about the duty to stand one's ground in the face of risk press as urgently upon the medical community today as ever (Battin et al., 2009; University of Toronto Joint Centre for Bioethics, 2005).

One standard way of thinking about these questions involves the notion of a social contract between the professions and society. On this view, health professions are forging a contract of sorts with the society at large. Those professions endorse and enforce a duty to provide care for the sick even in the face of personal risk, whereas society, for its part, grants to the health professions (and especially to physicians) social esteem, comfortable remuneration, and, perhaps most importantly, a great degree of professional autonomy, including the exclusive legal right to practice medicine. Perhaps the most powerful feature of this social contract argument is its recognition that if physicians, through licensure, are to be granted the exclusive legal prerogative of practicing medicine, then physicians must provide care to those in need even in the face of personal risk. If they do not provide care when at risk, and if the bargain physicians have struck with society denies to all other groups (e.g., herbalists, acupuncturists) the legal right to step in and do so, then no one will remain to care for the sick in times of great social need. It is difficult to imagine the effects, both for stricken individuals and for society at large, if health workers and hospitals refused to accept gravely ill and highly infectious patients.

A corollary of this line of thinking stresses the obligations that health professionals bear toward one another. If a front-line public health worker, physician, or nurse refuses to come into contact with sick and infectious patients, the latter will not simply disappear; they will inevitably become the charge of other health workers. The question, then, is not "Why me?," but rather, "If not me, then who?" If failure to care for patients in the presence of risk merely shifts the burden onto one's fellow health professionals, who must then shoulder even more than their fair share of risk, then such refusals amount to a serious injustice toward one's own colleagues.

An alternative approach to the duty to treat can be found in an ethic of virtue. According to this line of argument, the job of health workers is to attend to the needs of the sick. To do this job well, certain virtues are necessary, such as competence and courage in the face of adversity. Those who stress an appeal to the virtues as opposed to the social contract often respond, "This is who we are; this is what we do." Those who fail to exhibit some degree of courage in the face of personal risk are like firefighters who refuse to rescue people trapped in burning buildings or police officers who refuse to pursue suspected criminals down dark alleys. Confronting some degree of personal risk comes with the job of being a health worker. Those who refuse to run such risks arguably misunderstand what it means to be a doctor, nurse, or public health worker. The virtue orientation focuses attention squarely and directly on health professionals' mission of caring for those in need. The fact that this mission places such professionals in the path of personal risk lends it the aura of heroism and a higher calling—health professionals as civic guardians, not self-interested economic entrepreneurs.

The virtue perspective tends to focus on the individual health worker's ethical identity and responsibility, whereas the social contract perspective tends to focus on the duties of entire professions rather than on individual practitioners. Strictly speaking, the contractual duties of the medical profession to the larger society are theoretically compatible with a robust right of individual physicians to treat or refuse to treat whomever they wish. So long as a sufficient number of physicians remains on the job to care for those in need, others could opt out as they see fit. Although medical history is replete with examples of such opting out during times of plague, the virtue approach would view such examples as deviations from what should be expected from all health professionals, overriding their professional autonomy to pick and choose whom they wish to care for. The virtue approach also underscores the importance of inculcating requisite virtues into each new generation of physicians, nurses, and public health workers. Students should be aware that their chosen profession comes with various risks attached, so that one's eventual entry into such fields would presuppose a fully explicit acceptance of such hazards. Although such an acceptance was merely implicit, at best, during the period of the *pax antibiotica*, it must be fully explicit in a world threatened by AIDS, SARS, and pandemic influenza (World Health Organization, 2007).

Considered jointly, the social contract and virtue perspectives support a robust duty on the part of both the health professions collectively and health professionals individually to maintain their posts even in times of great social stress and threats of infectious disease. As elaborated so far, however, these complementary approaches may not be sufficient to account for three additional concerns: (1) What duties, if any, are owed by nonprofessionals providing health care and other emergency services? (2) What does the larger society owe to emergency workers? And (3), where should the line be drawn between professional duty (which is ethically mandatory) and what the philosophers call the realm of "supererogation," conduct above and beyond the call of duty (which is ethically discretionary)?

Regarding the first concern, one lesson of the recent SARS epidemic is that the burden of some infectious diseases might fall most heavily on hospitals, where the sickest and most infectious patients go for care and, in many cases, for isolation and quarantine. Although public health and health care professionals often heroically put themselves in harm's way, many nonprofessionals (including paramedics, radiographers, office workers, food service workers, and even janitorial staff) got sick, faced enormous psychological stress, and in some cases died during that epidemic (Knobler et al., 2004*b*). Whereas the health professionals (eventually) enjoyed enhanced public esteem and were in most cases provided with the requisite information and technical supports to protect themselves, the nonprofessionals faced similar risks without the luxury of choice or comparable access to social rewards, information, and protection (Reid, 2005). Now, assuming that the combined efforts of all these disparate professional and nonprofessional staff were necessary to keep the hospitals functioning in their battle against SARS, what can be said regarding the behavior of nonprofessionals during that crisis and possible future emergencies?

Neither the traditional social contract rationale nor the professional virtue approach sheds light on this question. Here, seeing emergency preparedness as a civic practice is helpful. The civic practice concept broadens the notion of a social contract between a profession and society because it focuses on function rather than credentials or specialized knowledge. It also leads to renewed appreciation for the duties of ordinary citizens to contribute to the common good during times of crisis. Seeing their role in civic practice would lead one to include administrators, food services personnel, and radiology technicians in the expanded social contract, but this would obviously call for a matching, broadened conception of the societal quid pro quo. Thus, in addition to the benefits of licensure, professional autonomy, and social esteem meted out to physicians, the equivalent of "battle pay," compensation for injury or death, and some appropriate form of public recognition could be envisioned for nonprofessional staffers.

Moreover, civic practice opens up the idea that threats posed to the social fabric on the order of SARS or pandemic influenza should engage the moral sensibilities not just of health professionals, but also of ordinary citizens who happen to serve as office workers and orderlies in hospitals and clinics. To subdue such threats to society, it could be argued that every member of the community must contribute what she or he can to the common effort; every oar must be in the water. Here, too, in order to avoid placing an undue burden on those members of the community who, because of their placement within the medical and public health infrastructures, face greater than average risks, public health planners would need to think of appropriate ways of honoring them and compensating them for their sacrifices.

What, then, does society owe to health workers? The notion of emergency preparedness as a civic practice—a broadened social contract—applies strongly to health workers, professionals and nonprofessionals alike. If health workers are willing to serve the needs of others and to face considerable risk in the line of duty, then society has a duty, especially in the context of an emergency, to provide them with the information and infection control measures and the protections and tools (training, equipment, supplies, security) they need to subdue the epidemic or blunt the effects of natural disasters. They should be supported both by society at large and government at all levels and also by local communities and health care institutions or other corporations that employ them. During the SARS outbreak, some of the physicians in China who refused to return to their hospitals did so precisely because they were outraged at what they perceived to be the government's ineptitude in handling the early stages of the epidemic and because they were afraid to engage with this mysterious new and lethal disease without adequate infection control protections (Brookes, 2005; Person et al., 2004).

Finally, there is a societal obligation associated with emergency preparedness to create and maintain an adequate infrastructure for public health. The focus here is systemic, not individual; it does not fall exclusively or even primarily on the virtues or expected sacrifices of individual health workers, but rather on our collective responsibility to provide and maintain an infrastructure conducive to their safety and the success of emergency preparedness and to routine, everyday public health. A well-funded and thoughtfully designed public health infrastructure is by far the best way for society to meet the wide array of currently unforeseeable threats and future emergencies. Narrowly targeted stockpiles and response plans for specific threats (e.g., hurricanes, anthrax, pandemic influenza) no doubt have their place; but they will most likely fail to achieve their objectives in the absence of a sound system of public health (see Chapter 2).

Society's ethical responsibility to health workers extends beyond material resources into the domain of social recognition, meaning, and self-esteem. There should be appropriate forms of social recognition for the sacrifices made by health workers. At a minimum, health workers should not be socially shunned, as many were during the Toronto SARS crisis. (Once it became known that health workers were transmitting that deadly disease, they were often shunned by the general public as potential carriers. Nurses in Toronto's hospitals reported that taxi drivers often refused to take them home from work.) More importantly, perhaps, society should strive to provide needed care to all health workers who become ill or disabled in the line of duty and to provide compensation to their families should they die (Huber & Wynia, 2004).

Now we come to the difficult question of how much risk health workers are morally and professionally obligated to accept in the context of a health emergency. Before discussing this question directly, two preliminary points should be noted.

First, any adequate accounting of the obligations borne by health care and public health professionals must acknowledge and take seriously the full complexity of their moral situation. The moral challenge here stems not simply from a potential conflict between professional duty and individuals' interest in avoiding serious morbidity and mortality, but also from health workers' competing moral obligations to their spouses or partners and children who depend on their support. This is not merely a question of self-centeredness but of divided ethical loyalties. It is not simply a test of moral will between self-interest and duty, where the right answer may be clear but difficult to follow. It is a genuine moral dilemma between competing moral obligations. In many cases, health workers might fear becoming ill and losing the ability to provide for their families; in others, they may be tempted to stay home in order to provide much-needed care to their own family members already stricken by disease or natural disaster (see Chapter 5).

Moreover, different sorts of disaster pose different levels of risk to health workers. A bioterrorist attack with chemicals or pathogens, for example, engenders widespread fear and panic in the general population, and especially in those living and working in close proximity to the event, but it does not ordinarily place health professionals working after the fact in a controlled environment at greatly increased personal risk. A major hurricane may not expose health workers to especially high levels of personal physical danger, but the psychosocial risks of working in such stressful conditions might pose a serious threat to their mental health (Tracy, 2007). (It is interesting to note that both Katrina and Sandy caused flooding and disruption of major hospitals and many nursing facilities. The siting, architecture, and construction design of health facilities is itself an element of emergency preparedness and future planning.) In certain extreme circumstances, such as the recent SARS epidemic or a predicted pandemic influenza crisis, health workers face very high risks of serious morbidity and mortality.

Unlike many infectious diseases, such as AIDS, which can be transmitted from person to person in the absence of symptoms, SARS became highly communicable only after patients had become sufficiently sick to become hospitalized. As a result, hospitals became places of infection and death, and many physicians and nurses died caring for SARS patients. Although the mortality rate for SARS worldwide hovered at the alarming average rate of 15%, health workers constituted a disturbingly large percentage of its victims at epicenters in Hong Kong (25%), Vietnam (100%), and Canada (65%). Those who did not become ill were nevertheless often quarantined in their hospitals for long periods of time, and many of these suffered greatly from the effects of isolation, including depression. Perhaps the most noteworthy thing about the SARS epidemic is that so many health workers showed up for work despite the alarming risks and the mysterious nature of the disease (Emanuel, 2003).

What, then, is the ethical answer to our third question? Medicine, nursing, and public health are inherently risky professions to some extent and always have been. Prior to heated debates over physicians' duty to treat HIV-infected patients during the late 1980s, health workers routinely treated, for example, psychiatry patients with violent tendencies and patients on tuberculosis wards. Indeed, one commentator argued at that time that physicians had a duty to treat AIDS patients because they had already accepted a certain level of risk by virtue of becoming physicians (Daniels, 1991). Since the risks posed by HIV were not significantly greater for physicians practicing adequate infection control than the background risks inherent in medical practice, the argument went that contemporary physicians can be assumed to have implicitly consented to treat patients with HIV.

On the other hand, no credible morality of medicine, nursing, or public health would impose a duty of martyrdom. Did Russian physicians have a duty to lower themselves by helicopter into the Chernobyl nuclear reactor to treat technicians exposed to fatal doses of radiation? In those desperate hours after the containment structure was breached, many workers and emergency responders, such as those shoveling debris and helicopter pilots trying to extinguish fires, did expose themselves knowingly to lethal radiation in order to contain the leakage and save lives. But, surely, in cases such as this, marked by extremely high levels of risk and inadequate protection, health workers do not have a moral or professional duty to treat. The public can always hope for heroic deeds, for health workers giving the last full measure of devotion, but it cannot expect or demand these things of doctors, nurses, or public health workers. Nor should health workers be expected to plunge into the fray without first having in place appropriate training, resources, protective equipment, and follow-up support to help perform their job safely. It is the duty of society at large (and health care institutions) to provide these resources. This is true in part because such workers have a duty to keep themselves healthy so that they can continue to treat others. Again, the provision of a robust public health infrastructure, including adequate personal protective equipment for health workers, not exhortations to heroism, should be the primary focus of emergency preparedness (Antares Foundation, 2006).

However, after acknowledging these points, the truly hard cases remain. Were the health workers who fell ill or died while caring for SARS patients just doing their duty, or did they transcend the call of duty into the realm of heroism, wherein we can be grateful to those who stood their ground but cannot criticize or condemn those who fled? Several commentators have pointed out that the remarkable thing about the SARS epidemic was the steadfastness of health professionals in the face of palpable and serious risk. The medical profession dithered, not to its credit, over its obligations to treat HIV-infected patients during the 1980s and 1990s (Arras, 1988). But physicians and other health workers by and large rose to the much more daunting challenge posed by SARS. It takes genuine courage for health workers to stand their ground in emergencies, and it is fitting and proper that they be honored for it. Students of nursing, medicine, and public health should be taught their names and told their stories.

Finally, the notion of professional duty should not be expected to do all the moral heavy lifting in this controversy. Health care and public health professionals have serious moral duties to serve the public good, even at reasonable risk to their life and health. However, society would be remiss if it concentrated solely on such duties to the exclusion of offering various incentives for altruistic behavior, especially when the level of risk begins to rise beyond the level of duty. In past epidemics, for example, cities have bestowed additional privileges or remuneration on "plague doctors" who stood their ground instead of fleeing, or bestowed licensure or guild privileges on practitioners who may not have been deemed eligible previously (Arras, 1988). Again, the most basic foundation for health professionals to answer an extraordinary call of duty is to ensure that institutional support and resources are in place, including, as mentioned earlier, appropriate training, resources, protective equipment, and follow-up support to help health personnel perform their job safely. Additional support to ensure that the health care workforce responds in an emergency might include such things as increased pay; the reliable backup of specialized hospital units well stocked with highly skilled practitioners, technology, and medications; giving first-responders high priority in the distribution of scarce vaccines and prophylactic medications; and special supports for ill family members. If health care and public health professionals can be reassured that their ill family members will be properly cared for, their moral dilemma will be attenuated, which will make it easier for them to assume their proper posts at the barricades.

Civic Obligations and Personal Responsibility

Albert Camus wrote, “What’s true of all the evils in the world is true of the plague as well. It helps men to rise above themselves” (Camus, 1991). And indeed, one important dimension of emergency preparedness is to foster a sense of civic obligation and a concern for the well-being of the community as a whole on the part of all citizens and community residents. A closely related goal is to prepare individuals and families to understand what their responsibilities will be during an emergency and to equip them with information and possibly other resources to react appropriately and responsibly at such a time. These goals are both ethical and practical. The discussion in this section relates to the ethical goal of promoting personal and civic responsibility, but it also relates to the goal of developing resilient and just, as well as safe communities. Public health professionals and other leaders should use the planning process to strengthen the social capital of communities and to make them more resilient so that they can weather all hazards and emergencies—which are now inevitable throughout the globe and no community is immune from them—with as little damage as possible and bounce back from emergencies quickly and return to civic health (Barbee, 2007; Erikson, 1976, 1994; Paton & Johnston, 2006; Vale & Campanella, 2005).

Here, we return to the distinction we have drawn between the civic and the consumerist models of emergency preparedness. Recall that, through the lens of the consumer model, emergency planning is rather like medical or financial planning. Providers with specialized knowledge are preparing a product for clients who are using that product to promote their own interests as consumers.

From a civic perspective, emergency planning is not a commodity to be exchanged between a consumer with an interest and a provider with the expertise to fulfill that interest. It is a public function, a part of the basic purpose of forming a political community in the first place: the security, life, liberty, and well-being of the people as a whole (Benjamin, 2006). It is not the property of those who create it; it is not simply "used" by those who benefit from it. It is an expression of the entire community about the value of the lives and health of its members (Honig, 2009). It is a covenant of public trust, an agreement to be entered into by all that establishes commitments of responsibility for each.

Moreover, a growing body of public health and epidemiologic research is demonstrating that the health status of individuals is not merely a function of their genetic makeup, their biological functioning, and the toxic substances or microorganisms they are exposed to in their physical and biological environment. Physical health, to say nothing of mental health and psychological well-being, is affected by the sociocultural environment (Berkman & Kawachi, 2000; Daniels, Kennedy, & Kawachi, 1999; Evans, Marer, & Marmor, 1994; Frumkin et al., 2004; Marmot, 2004; Putnam, 2000; Wilkinson, 1996; Wilkinson & Pickett, 2009). Everyday health risk factors associated with the breakdown or absence of civic resources (so-called *social capital*) are also risk factors pertinent to what will happen during emergency situations. The capacity of individuals to respond and the capacity of communities to respond are interrelated. Each factor separately, as well their complex (if still poorly understood) interrelationship, should be of central interest and concern to the emergency planner.

Fostering Civic and Personal Responsibility

The fact that emergency preparedness is primarily a societal and a governmental responsibility does not obviate the fact that there are significant moral obligations incumbent on private citizens as well. The previous section addressed the special obligations attendant on the role of "professionals" in society, in particular health professionals. This section views each person in his or her dual identity as democratic citizen and as a private moral agent. By "citizen," we mean not so much a legal status, but the ethical and social role of being a responsible member of a political community of free and equal persons, a community of reciprocal rights and obligations, a community of shared vulnerability and risk, and a community of mutual concern and respect. By viewing persons as private "moral agents," we bring to the foreground their personal, as distinct from their civic, lives: that is, their web of familial and kinship relationships, friendships, and personal associations.

Earlier, we discussed the importance of building active voice and involvement for citizens in the planning process. Doing this is supported by considerations of rights and respect, ensuring justice and nondiscrimination, and making an emergency plan more intelligent and effective by tapping into the kinds of local knowledge that experts may overlook. An added dimension of this process is that undertaking planning and the other activities that mitigate community vulnerability to hazards and that strengthen the community's resilience will engage people in ways that renew or strengthen their own sense of civic responsibility and membership (Barbee, 2007). It may also reinforce the health of those organizations of neighborhood and civil society that make up the infrastructure of civic life and are integral to the ability to recover from disaster and dislocation (Hoffman & Oliver-Smith, 2002; Pelling, 2003; Savitch, 2008).

An example of this was demonstrated in the village of Shang-An in Taiwan. In 2001, Taiwan, a country prone to recurrent public health and weather-related emergency events, began efforts to improve the country's emergency response capability and to explore ways in which people at the grassroots level can be integrated into the preparedness and planning process. In Shang-An, public engagement activities demonstrated how "street science" can be used as residents shared their knowledge of local ecology, terrain, and other conditions. They became a part of a kind of surveillance and early warning system. They also formed effective community organizations to take an active role in problem-solving and in undertaking hazard mitigation and emergency management tasks (Chen, Lui, & Chan, 2006).

Having the opportunity to take part in such local, community-based public health functions has an educational effect on citizens and helps to promote greater scientific and health literacy. This in turn spills over the line between peoples' sense of communal membership and civic responsibility as citizens and their sense of responsibility for the health and safety of themselves and their families as moral agents (Schafer et al., 2008). By taking part in emergency preparedness and hazard mitigation efforts, a person can bring closer together the civic and the personal realms of his or her life and conscience. Not only will vulnerability to various public health hazards be thereby mitigated, but so too will the radical privatization and the alienation from the civic realm that so many who "bowl alone" in America now apparently feel.[13] When large numbers of volunteers show up at an emergency site to help, we may always admire their expression of solidarity and mutual concern, but we need not forever be astounded by it (Solnit, 2009).

We believe that a sense of citizen obligations, concern for the common good, and a sense of personal and familial responsibility generally reinforce one another. However, there may be times when a conflict of obligations seems to arise. Certainly, most compelling moral obligations during a time of threat or crisis are those obligations of moral agency that pertain to a person's role as parent, spouse, relative, or friend. And, of course, private individuals have rights and duties that pertain to themselves, in particular, the right to self-preservation.

Here, we address such conflicts between civic and the personal duties: how to prevent, avoid, and mitigate them as much as possible through the pre-event planning process and, if they do arise, how to think through and resolve them.

Emergency Preparedness and Private Dilemmas

It is important not to carry the notion of fusion of public and private, civic responsibility and personal responsibility too far. When this is done, communal conformity can eclipse individuality, privacy, and the liberty that leads to diversity. Ethical conflicts and dilemmas will undoubtedly arise in the context of emergency preparedness. Plans tell people how to behave in the face of impending danger, but people ultimately have to take responsibility for how prudently and responsibly they act to protect themselves and their families. Private moral agency and personal responsibility wrestle with scarcities of various kinds, and these scarcities become dramatic in the emergency preparedness context.

Everyone should be informed about steps they can take to prepare for an emergency and what to do to find shelter, to evacuate, or to locate medical care. Much information regarding these things is now available, although some reports suggest that it is being conveyed in ways that are not sensitive to ethnic or class differences (Falkheimer & Heide, 2006; James et al., 2007). It is not obvious, for example, that prudence and private moral responsibility dictate that more immediate needs (rent, children's clothing, education) should be forgone so that one can stock up a 90-day supply of canned goods. Public health emergency planning should assume a measure of self-protection and personal responsibility on the part of ordinary people, and it should give them the information they need to make informed choices. However, emergency planning must also accommodate the reality of limited choices and resources that many people confront in their normal lives, for these will constrain them before, during, and after an emergency as well. Emergency preparedness plans should not take for granted or require undue burden or self-sacrifice. A just society will provide adequate social provision so that mothers and fathers will be able to make prudent individual provision for the health and safety of their family without making tragic tradeoffs (Powers & Faden, 2006).

No one can be in two places at the same time, and physical presence can take on an importance in times of crisis that it does not in everyday life. What do we say about the man who was in his office when the plane hit Tower 1 of the World Trade Center and who decided to search the floor for survivors rather than go immediately to the stairway to escape and protect himself? What does one say to his wife and children? Perhaps he had a special task in case of fire in the evacuation plan that his agency had prepared some time ago. Should he—or should anyone—have accepted that role and that responsibility? Yet if no one does, if no one should, how can there ever be any emergency plan?

Recommendations on Ethical Emergency Planning

When considering particular aspects of an emergency plan or policies that will govern the response to emergency situations, public health officials and other stakeholders can be realistically guided by well-established aspects of sound ethical analysis and decision making (Kass, 2001, 2004, 2005). They can also be guided by the civic values and goals of preparedness planning and of public health generally. The purpose of giving this attention to ethics is to make emergency preparedness planners alert to a broad range of values, keep them attentive to the types of factual information that bear on ethical decisions or value judgments, and encourage them to remain flexible and open to diverse points of view while still confident and decisive enough in their judgments to meet the challenges of advance planning and emergency response situations.

To supplement the recommendations made elsewhere in the literature of public health ethics and in other chapters in this volume, we propose that ethically responsible public health planners adopt the following practices:

1. *Be clear about the goals of a proposed emergency response intervention or mitigation.*[14] Identify its goals and ascertain that these goals are consonant with the widely accepted goals and objectives of the public health profession. For example, a proposed emergency response that gives priority to protection of property over protection of human life and health should be subject to special scrutiny and would require special

justification. This is a stark example, but it is not entirely hypothetical. As was observed in New Orleans in the aftermath of Hurricane Katrina and massive flooding, officials were so concerned about looting that they devoted scarce financial and manpower resources to law enforcement and security activities while rescue, evacuation, and other health measures were being inadequately supported.

2. *Be sure that a proposed emergency response intervention is based on the most reliable factual information that is reasonably available to decision-makers under the circumstances.* Identify and assess the available factual information. In making this assessment, planners should be careful to weigh the evidence indicating that the proposed emergency response will be effective in attaining its goals. They also should not jump to conclusions or fail to consider a range of alternatives. Emergency public health planning will always have to wrestle with the reliability, the completeness, and the timeliness of the information available to it. There is no such thing as perfect information, but that does not mean that decision-makers do not have a responsibility to use the best information they have. Arbitrary and ill-informed decisions are not ethically acceptable, even in emergency situations.
3. *Be aware of the ethical values that are affected (promoted or undermined) by the proposed emergency response and by the ways in which it is carried out.* Values may be defined as those states of affairs that promote human flourishing. Almost by definition, public health will promote the values of human life, safety, and health. However, emergency response activities encroach into an ethical domain that is broader than specific public health values alone. Therefore, in an ethical assessment of a proposed emergency response, it is important to be aware of values concerning liberty, justice and equality, dignity, respect, responsible stewardship of scarce resources, transparency and accountability, maintaining public trust, and professional integrity (Thomas, Sage, Dillenberg, & Guillory, 2002).

When planners take ethical values seriously they ask the following kinds of questions:

- How can the plan best achieve public health effectiveness with minimal coercion?
- Among available alternatives, which emergency response is most efficient?
- Which alternative is the least harmful and burdensome?
- Are important individual rights or interests going to be sacrificed for health and safety?
- Will the emergency response have effects that are fair and equitable; in other words, will the benefits and burdens caused by the planned emergency response be distributed justly across the affected population?
- Can the emergency response be implemented in a respectful and nondiscriminatory fashion?

4. *Be concrete rather than abstract in ethical thinking; put a face on the individuals and groups who will be most directly affected by a proposed emergency response intervention.* One way to do this is to perform an assessment that will identify the "stakeholders" in a decision. Stakeholders may be defined as those whose rights or interests are significantly affected by a decision. Special efforts should be made to include and to consider the interests of vulnerable or marginalized stakeholders who may not have the power to influence the decision unless special provision is made to ensure their participation. For example, stakeholder assessment asks: Who will benefit from the proposed emergency response? Who will be burdened by it? Who should have a voice in making the decision?
5. *Be aware that the process of decision-making leading up to the selection of an emergency response can raise important ethical considerations in its own right.* Many times, people are so focused on content (what is to be decided) that they do not become self-consciously analytic and critical about process (how it is to be decided). But it is ethically important to consider the process for making the decision and the values that pertain to the process—participation, inclusiveness, public

and open deliberation, fair hearings, adequate technical support and expertise. It is also important for emergency preparedness planners to consider the institutional properties of the decision-making process itself: it should be designed with checks and balances, redundancy, feedback loops for learning from mistakes and for making mid-course corrections, and an appeals process to review decisions that come under challenge. The types of questions that should be asked are: Is the decision-making process fairly representative and inclusive? Is it open and transparent? Is it intelligently responsive: that is, does the implementation process include the capacity to monitor and evaluate progress and to learn from mistakes or unanticipated consequences?

6. *Take steps to enable careful evaluation of the emergency response later. How will public health planners know if an emergency response is successful, has met its goals, has been implemented ethically, and has had good ethical effects?* This brings the process full circle, since having clearly defined and stated goals at the outset is a prerequisite for proper evaluation later on. For example, ask such questions as: What are our criteria of evaluation? Are data being gathered or records being kept such that it will be possible to conduct an evaluation and assessment of the emergency response later?
7. *Be aware of and resist unwarranted urgency in implementing an emergency response.* Consider the timing of the emergency response in an analytic way. Avoid the exaggeration of risk and worst-case scenarios. Resist precipitous action. This is particularly important if one feels that the ethical analysis of a proposed emergency response is inadequate or incomplete. Of course, excessive caution, weak resolve, and procrastination are undesirable and often harmful as well. Leaders and decision-makers have difficult judgments to make, and what is needed is perhaps the ethical equivalent of "due diligence." For example, ask questions such as the following: Why exactly does this decision have to be made immediately? Is there time for the collection of additional information or data without

taking undue risk? Is there time for broader community consultation before a final decision has to be made, particularly if very difficult and consequential ethical decisions have to be made?

Conclusion

Emergency preparedness is a vital public health function. As such, it is both a governmental responsibility and a civic endeavor. This chapter has presented a broad overview of its subject, as opposed to a focused look at one aspect of emergency preparedness, such as the response to pandemic influenza, bioterrorism, or weather-related emergencies. The purpose of this chapter has been to provide an ethically orientating perspective on emergency preparedness understood as a complex practice or activity with intrinsic values and standards of competency. Society needs such an orientation and a rich, ethical vocabulary, capable of expressing nuance, pluralism, and a commitment to responsible democratic citizenship and the common good.

We believe that there is considerable value in providing resources for ongoing, serious conversation and deliberation about ethics. There is much that is not yet understood about how to do emergency planning and preparedness well. The epidemiologic, clinical, and behavioral sciences are still on a learning curve in the field. Likewise, there is still much to be learned about the ethics of what Elaine Scarry (2011) calls, "thinking in emergencies."

Emergency preparedness is ultimately not only about protecting a population. It is also about sustaining and building or rebuilding civic community and strengthening it. Successful emergency planning must rely on and tap into a preexisting fund of civic responsibility, a sense of justice, and concern for others in need. Emergency planning can and should be an occasion to foster these outlooks and impulses as well. Fear and self-interest will no doubt be strongly in evidence during any public health emergency, but public health leadership, in conjunction with elected officials and other community leaders, can move communities beyond these motivations to a sense of common purpose and solidarity. If it does this, public health emergency preparedness and response will succeed in meeting its ethical obligations and will most likely succeed in its practical efforts as well.

Notes

1. For a comprehensive review of emergency plans worldwide and the literature on emergency planning, see the work of Angela Witt Prehn and Dorothy E. Vawter (2008).

2. The paradigm of emergency preparedness that provides the most latitude for achieving high ethical standards and ideals is a broad social model of emergency planning. It brings public health into contact with similarly oriented perspectives and movements in cognate fields. It draws orientation from social epidemiology and "place-based" (ecosystem landscape and built environment) public health, community-based participatory research, deliberative planning, and the building of "learning communities" and "learning organizations" in management and leadership science (Forester, 1999; Schön & Rein, 1997). It may even have an analogue in law enforcement and criminal justice theories of community policing (Friedmann & Cannon, 2007).

3. What is the conceptual import of the concept of "resilience," and what are its implications for public health preparedness? A resilient community is not simply one that is able to "bounce back" or "rebound" to the status quo ante. This is the sense of resilience prevalent in psychology and medicine. However, in ecology and related fields, resilience is the capacity of a (natural or social) system to absorb external disturbances without losing its essential continuity and coherence (Adger, 2000; Gunderson & Holling, 2002; Walker & Salt, 2006). Building the second conception of resilience capacity into public health emergency planning opens up new possibilities for linking the underlying vitality and integrity of communities and systems of social capital with the concepts of "preparedness" and "security." As we use the term here, resilience is the capacity of a community (and of the individuals who comprise it) to respond creatively, preventatively, and proactively to change or extreme events, thus mitigating crisis

or disaster. In the emergency preparedness context, we focus especially on the social or community dimension of the concept. Social resilience is defined by Adger as "the ability of groups or communities to cope with external stresses and disturbances as a result of social, political and environmental change. This definition highlights social resilience in relation to the concept of ecological resilience which is a characteristic of ecosystems to maintain themselves in the face of disturbance" (Adger, 2000). Resilient communities have robust internal support systems and networks of mutual assistance and solidarity. They also maintain sustainable and risk mitigating relationships with their local ecosystems and their natural environment (Middaugh, 2008; Walker & Salt, 2006). Public health professionals and other leaders should use the preparedness planning process to empower communities by strengthening their social capital and to make them more resilient, so that they can weather all hazards and emergencies—which are now inevitable throughout the globe and no community is immune from them—with as little damage as possible, recover from disasters effectively, and return to civic health.

4. Berlin then continues: "To threaten a man with persecution unless he submits to a life in which he exercises no choices of his goals; to block before him every door but one, no matter how noble the prospect upon which it opens, or how benevolent the motives of those who arrange this, is to sin against the truth that he is a man, a being with a life of his own to live . . . I wish to be the instrument of my own, not of other men's, acts of will. I wish to be a subject, not an object; to be moved by reasons, by conscious purposes, which are my own, not by causes which affect me, as it were, from outside" (Berlin, 1969, p. 127).

5. Here, we follow the standard meaning of this term in economics, where the "opportunity cost" of any given public expenditure, *x*, is the value of those alternative opportunities society must forgo because of a decision to spend money on *x* rather than on those other things.

6. For information on current stockpiling goals and procedures, see http://www.bt.cdc.gov/stockpile/.

7. For an analogous example of this kind of thinking, one prominent public official has opined that, in the context of the post-9/11 world, "if there's a one percent chance that Pakistani scientists are helping al Qaeda build or develop a nuclear weapon, we have to treat it as a certainty in terms of our response" (Sunstein, 2007).

8. The Maginot Line was a chain of defensive fortifications built by France on its eastern border between World War I and World War II. It was designed to stop any future invasion by Germany; in World War II, the Germans conquered France by going around the Maginot Line to the north.

9. Generally speaking, during evacuation events, recalcitrant adults are permitted to make their own decisions to leave or to remain in place. If it is a toxic gas release, and an immediate threat to life was in the balance, perhaps no one would choose to stay, thus making coercive removal unnecessary; or, arguably, the imminent threat to life would more easily justify paternalistic coercion and forcible removal. Yet another dimension of complexity arises in the case of minor or incompetent adults. Should parents or guardians have the right to endanger such persons by refusing evacuation? Moreover, one's intuitions and judgments may vary as one considers infectious disease events and social distancing measures rather than evaluation events. This suggests that the specific context and circumstances matter in emergency preparedness ethics. Nonetheless, more research is needed on circumstances involving harm to children and other dependents, and clearer standards on the limits of parental and guardian authority would be helpful. Here, public health ethics and public health law overlap and might well work in collaboration to develop such standards.

10. There is some disagreement about the definition of the term "transparency." For some, open meeting and open records requirements are sufficient to provide transparency in the operation of some decision-making body. We understand transparency to require at least some measure of justification and explanation: not just telling people after the fact what has been decided but attempting to explain why it has been decided. Transparency also requires that the public be provided with the necessary education, background information, and resources to intelligently assess what they are being told and what has been decided or proposed.

11. Current information concerning the Model Act and state legislative activity pertaining to it can be found on the website of the Johns Hopkins University and Georgetown University Centers for Law and the Public's Health at http://www.publichealthlaw.net/ModelLaws/MSEHPA.php.

12. The metaphor of a ladder of intervention is used by the Nuffield Council on Bioethics (2007) to convey the sequence of public health measures from the least to the most restrictive of individual liberty.

13. The phrase refers to a study by the sociologist Robert Putnam (2000) of the decline of civic engagement in America, including declining participation in social bowling leagues.

14. When we refer to "proposed" emergency responses or interventions, we certainly intend to suggest that ethical assessment should take place prior to making a decision or carrying out an emergency preparedness policy or response. But this does not preclude the important role of ethical analysis as an ongoing part of the entire emergency preparedness cycle. Ethical considerations can help to make mid-course corrections during the hours, days, or weeks of the response phase. Ethical considerations can also be helpful retrospectively so that emergency preparedness can learn from past mistakes and improve over time.

References

Adger, W. N. (2000). Social and ecological resilience: Are they related? *Progress in Human Geography*, *24*, 347–64.

Agamben, G. (2005). *State of exception (translated by Kevin Attell)*. Chicago: University of Chicago Press.

Altevogt, B. M., Stroud, C., Nadig, L., & Hougan, M (Rapporteurs). (2010). *Medical surge capacity: Workshop summary. Institute of Medicine Forum on Medical and Public Health Preparedness for Catastrophic Events, Board on Health Sciences Policy*. Washington, DC: National Academies Press. Available at http://www.nap.edu/download.php?record_id=12798.

Annas, G. J. (2002). Bioterrorism, public health, and civil liberties. *New England Journal of Medicine*, *346*, 1337–1342.

Annas, G. J., Mariner, W. K., & Parmet, W. E. (2008). *Pandemic preparedness: The need for a public health–not a law enforcement/national security approach*. New York: American Civil Liberties Union. Available at http://www.aclu.org/privacy/medical/33642pub20080114.html.

Antares Foundation. (2006). *Managing stress in humanitarian workers: Guidelines for good practice*. Amsterdam, Netherlands: Author.

Arras, J. D. (1988). The fragile web of responsibility: AIDS and the duty to treat. *Hastings Center Report, 18*, 10–20.

Arras, J. D. (2006). Rationing vaccine during an avian influenza pandemic: Why it won't be easy. *Yale Journal of Biology and Medicine, 78*, 287–300.

Baker, R. B., Caplan, A. L., & Latham, S. (1999). *The American medical ethics revolution: How the AMA's code of ethics has transformed physicians' relationships to patients, professionals and society*. Baltimore, M. D.: John Hopkins University Press.

Barbee, D. (2007). Disaster response and recovery: Strategies and tactics for resilience. *Journal of Homeland Security and Emergency Management, 4*(1), ISSN (Online) 1547-7355, DOI: 10.2202/1547-7355.1323, March.

Barnes M. D., Novilla, L. M. B., Meacham, A. T., McIntyre, E., & Erickson, B. C. (2008). Analysis of media agenda setting during and after Hurricane Katrina: Implications for emergency preparedness, disaster response, and disaster policy. *American Journal of Public Health, 98*, 604–610.

Battin, P. P., Francis, L. P., Jacobson, J. A., & Smith, C. B. (2009). *The patient as victim and vector: Ethics and infectious disease*. New York: Oxford University Press.

Bayer, R., & Fairchild, A. L. (2004). The genesis of public health ethics. *Bioethics, 18*, 473–492.

Benjamin, C. G. (2006). Putting the public in public health: New approaches. *Health Affairs, 25*, 1040–1043.

Berkman L. F., & Kawachi, I. (2000). *Social epidemiology*. Oxford: Oxford University Press.

Berlin, I. (1969). *Four essays on liberty*. Oxford: Oxford University Press.

Bodenheimer, T. (1997). The Oregon health plan—Lessons for the nation. *New England Journal of Medicine, 337*, 651–656.

Brock, D. (2004). Ethical issues in the use of cost effectiveness analysis for the prioritization of health care resources. In S. Anand, A. Peter, & A. Sen (Eds.), *Public health, ethics and equity* (pp. 201–223). Oxford: Oxford University Press.

Bröckling, U., Krasmann, S., & Lemke, T. (Eds.). (2010). *Govermentality: Current issues and future challenges*. New York: Routledge.

Brookes, T. J. & Kahn, O. A. (2005). *Behind the mask: How the world survived SARS*. Washington, DC: American Public Health Association.

Buchanan, D. R. (2000). *An ethic for health promotion: Rethinking the sources of human well-being*. New York: Oxford University Press.

Bytheway, B. (2006). The evacuation of older people: The case of Hurricane Katrina. In *Understanding Katrina: Perspectives from the social sciences*. Social Science Research Council. Available at http://understandingkatrina.ssrc.org/Bytheway/.

Calabresi, G., & Bobbitt, P. (1978). *Tragic choices*. New York: W. W. Norton.

Campion, E. W. (1999). Liberty and the control of tuberculosis. *New England Journal of Medicine, 340*, 385–386.

Camus, A. (1991). *The plague*. New York: Vintage Books.

Carter-Pokras, O., Zambrana R. E., Mora S. E., & Aaby K. A. (2007). Emergency preparedness: Knowledge and perceptions of Latin American immigrants. *Journal of the Poor and Underserved, 18*, 465–481.

Center for Health and the Global Environment. (2005). *Climate change futures: Health, ecological and economic dimensions*. Boston: Harvard Medical School. Available at http://coralreef.noaa.gov/aboutcrcp/strategy/reprioritization/wgroups/resources/climate/resources/cc_futures.pdf.

Center for Law and the Public's Health. (2001). The model state emergency health powers act. Georgetown University and Johns Hopkins University. Available at http://www.publichealthlaw.net/M. S.. E.HPA/M. S.. E.HPA2.pdf.

Chambers, S. (2003). Deliberative democratic theory. *Annual Review of Political Science, 6*, 307–318.

Chen, L. C., Lui Y. C., & Chan K. C. (2006). Integrated community-based disaster management program in Taiwan: A case study of Shang-An Village. *Journal of Natural Hazards, 37*, 209–223.

Childress J. F., & Bernheim R. G. (2003). Beyond the liberal and communitarian impasse: A framework and vision for public health. *Florida Law Review, 55*(5), 1191–1231.

Conly, S. (2013). *Against autonomy: Justifying coercive paternalism*. Cambridge: Cambridge University Press.

Cooper, C., & Block, R. (2006). *Disaster: Hurricane Katrina and the failure of homeland security*. New York: Times Books.

Corburn, J. (2005). *Community knowledge and environmental health justice*. Cambridge, MA: MIT Press.

Daniels, N. (1991). Duty to treat or right to refuse? *Hastings Center Report*, *21*, 36–46.

Daniels, N., Kennedy, B. P., & Kawachi, I. (1999). Why justice is good for our health: The social determinants of health inequalities. *Daedalus*, *128*, 215–51.

Daniels, N., Kettl, D. F., & Kunreuther, H. (2006). *On risk and disaster: Lessons from Hurricane Katrina*. Philadelphia, PA: University of Philadelphia Press.

Daniels, N., & Sabin, J. (2002). *Setting limits fairly*. Oxford: Oxford University Press.

Davis, E., & Mincin, J. (2006). *Incorporating special needs populations into emergency planning and exercises. Nobody left behind: Disaster preparedness for persons with mobility impairment*. Lawrence: University of Kansas, Research and Training Center on Independent Living.

DeBruin, D. A., Parilla, E., Liaschenko, J., Marshall, M. F., Leider J. P., Brunnquell, D., . . . Vawter, D. E. (2010). *Implementing ethical frameworks for rationing scarce health resources in Minnesota during severe influenza pandemic*. Minneapolis: University of Minnesota Center for Bioethics and Minnesota Center for Health Care Ethics.

Drexel University Center for Health Equality. (2008). *National consensus statement on integrating racially and ethnically diverse communities into public health emergency preparedness*. Washington, DC: US Department of Health and Human Services, Office of Minority Health.

Dworkin, R. (1993). *Life's dominion*. New York: Knopf.

Elder, K. A., Xirasagar, S., Miller, N., Bowen, S. A., Glover, S., & Piper, C. (2007). African Americans' decisions not to evacuate New Orleans before Hurricane Katrina: A qualitative study. *American Public Health Association*, *97*(Suppl 1), S124–S129.

Emanuel, E. J. (2003). The lessons of SARS. *Annals of Internal Medicine*, *139*, 589–591.

Erikson, K. T. (1976). *Everything in its path: Destruction of community in the Buffalo Creek flood*. New York: Simon and Schuster.

Erikson, K. T. (1994). *A new species of trouble: The human experience of modern disasters*. New York: W. W. Norton.

Evans, R. G., Marer, M. L., & Marmor, T. R. (1994). *Why are some people healthy and others not?* New York: Aldine de Gruyter.

Fain, B., Viswanathan, K., & Altevogt, B. M. (Rapporteurs). (2012). *Public engagement on facilitating access to antiviral medications and information in an influenza pandemic: Workshop series summary*. Institute of Medicine Forum on Medical and Public Health Preparedness for Catastrophic Events, Board on Health Sciences Policy. Washington, DC: National Academies Press. Available at www.nap.edu/download.php?record_id=13404.

Fairchild, A. L., Colgrove, J., & Jones, M. M. (2006). The challenge of mandatory evacuation: Providing for and deciding for. *Health Affairs*, *25*, 958–967.

Falkheimer, J., & Heide, M. (2006). Multicultural crisis communication: Toward a social constructionist perspective. *Journal of Contingencies and Crisis Management*, *14*, 180–189.

Fleck, L. M. (2009). *Just caring: Health care rationing and democratic deliberation*. New York: Oxford University Press.

Forester, J. (1999). *The deliberative practitioner: Encouraging participatory planning processes*. Cambridge, MA: MIT Press.

Frankel, M. S. (1989). Professional codes: Why, how, and with what impact? *Journal of Business Ethics*, *8*, 109–115.

Frickel, S. (2006). Our toxic gumbo: Recipe for a politics of environmental knowledge. In *Understanding Katrina: Perspectives from the social sciences*. Social Science Research Council. Available at http://understandingkatrina.ssrc.org/Frickel/.

Friedman, A. (2008). Beyond accountability for reasonableness. *Bioethics*, *22*, 101–112.

Friedmann, R. R., & Cannon, W. J. (2007). Homeland security and community policing: Competing or complementing public safety policies. *Journal of Homeland Security and Emergency Management*, *4*(4), ISSN (Online) 1547-7355, DOI: 10.2202/1547-7355.1371, December 2007.

Frumkin, H., Frank, L., & Jackson, R. (2004). *Urban sprawl and public health: Designing, planning, and building for healthy communities*. Washington, DC: Island Press.

Frumkin, H., & McMichael A. J. (2008). Climate change and public health: Thinking, communicating, acting, *American Journal of Preventive Medicine*, *35*(5), 403–410.

Fussell, E. (2006). Leaving New Orleans: Social stratification, networks, and hurricane evacuation. In *Understanding Katrina: Perspectives from the social sciences*. Social Science Research Council. Available at http://understandingkatrina.ssrc.org/Fussell/.

Garrett, J. E., Vawter, D. E., Gervais, K. G., Prehn, A. W., DeBruin, D. A., Livingston, F., . . . Lynfield, R. (2011). The Minnesota pandemic ethics project: Sequenced, robust public engagement process. *Journal of Participatory Medicine, 3*(e6). Available from: http://www.jopm.org/evidence/research/2011/01/19/the-minnesota-pandemic-ethics-project-sequenced-robust-public-engagement-processes/.

Garrett, J. E., Vawter, D. E., Prehn, A. W., DeBruin, D. A., & Gervais K. G. (2008). Ethical considerations in pandemic influenza planning. *Minnesota Medicine, 91*(4), 37–39.

Garrett, J. E., Vawter, D. E., Prehn, A. W., DeBruin, D. A., & Gervais, K. G. (2009). Listen! The value of public engagement in pandemic ethics. *American Journal of Bioethics, 9*(11), 17–19.

Gaylin, W., & Jennings, B. (2003). *The perversion of autonomy: Coercion and constraints in a liberal society* (2nd edition). Washington, DC: Georgetown University Press.

Gilman, N. (2006). What Katrina teaches about the meaning of racism. In *Understanding Katrina: Perspectives from the social sciences*. Social Science Research Council. Available at http://understandingkatrina.ssrc.org/Gilman/.

Goodin, R. (1995). *Utilitarianism as a public philosophy*. New York: Cambridge University Press.

Gostin, L. O. (2003). When terrorism threatens health: how far are limitations on human rights justified? *Florida Law Review, 55*, 1105–1170.

Gostin, L. O., Sapsin, J. W., Teret, S. P., Burris, S., Mair, J. S., Hodge, J. R., Jr., & Vernick, J. S. (2002). The model state emergency health powers act: Planning for and response to bioterrorism and naturally occurring infectious diseases. *Journal of the American Medical Association, 288*, 622.

Gould, S. D., Biddle, A. K., Klipp, G., Hall, C. N., & Danis, M. (2005). Choosing health plans all together: A deliberative exercise for allocating limited health care resources. *Journal of Health Politics, Policy and Law, 30*, 563–601.

Graham, S. (2006). Cities under siege: Katrina and the politics of metropolitan America. In *Understanding Katrina: Perspectives from the social sciences*. Social Science Research Council. Available at http://understandingkatrina.ssrc.org/Graham/.

Gunderson, L. H., & Holling, C. S. (Eds.) (2002). *Panarchy: Understanding transformation in human and natural systems*. Washington: Island Press.

Gutmann, A., & Thompson, D. (1996). *Democracy and disagreement*. Cambridge, MA: Harvard University Press.

Hanfling, D., Altevogt, B. M., Viswanathan, K., & Gostin, L. O. (Eds.). (2012). *Crisis standards of care: A systems framework for catastrophic disaster response*. Institute of Medicine, Committee on Guidance for Establishing Crisis Standards of Care for Use in Disaster Situations. Washington, DC: National Academies Press. Available at http://www.nap.edu/download.php?record_id=13351.

Hartman, C., & Squires G. D. (2006). *There is no such thing as a natural disaster: Race, class, and Hurricane Katrina*. New York: Routledge.

Health Systems Research Inc. (2005). *Altered standards of care in mass casualty events*. Report No. 05–0043. Washington, DC: Agency for Healthcare Research and Quality.

Hoffman, S. M., & Oliver-Smith, A. (2002). *Catastrophe and culture: The anthropology of disaster*. Santa Fe, NM: School of American Research Press.

Holland, S. (2007). *Public health ethics*. Cambridge: Polity Press.

Honig, B. (2009). *Emergency politics: Paradox, law, democracy*. Princeton, NJ: Princeton University Press.

Huber, S. J., & Wynia, M. K. (2004). When pestilence prevails: Physician responsibilities in epidemics. *American Journal of Bioethics, 4*, W5–W11.

Institute of Medicine. (2003). *The future of the public's health in the 21st century*. Washington, DC: National Academies Press.

Institute of Medicine. Committee on implementation of antiviral medication strategies for an influenza pandemic. (2008). *Antivirals for pandemic influenza: Guidance on developing a distribution and dispensing program*. Washington: National Academies Press.

James, X., Hawkins, A., & Rowel, R. (2007). An assessment of the cultural appropriateness of emergency preparedness communication for low income minorities. *Journal of Homeland Security and Emergency Management*, *4*(3), ISSN (Online) 1547-7355, DOI: 10.2202/1547-7355.1266, September 2007.

Jennings, B. (2003). On authority and justification in public health. *Florida Law Review*, *55*, 1241–1256.

Jennings, B. (2007a). Community in public health ethics. In R. E. Ashcroft, A. Dawson, H. Draper, & J. McMillan (Eds.), *Principles of health care ethics*. West Sussex: Wiley.

Jennings, B. (2007b). Public health and civic republicanism. In A. Dawson & M. Verweij (Eds.), *Ethics, prevention, and public health*. Oxford: Oxford University Press.

Jensen, E. (Ed.). (1997). *Disaster management ethics*. United Nations Department of Humanitarian Affairs and the Disaster Management Training Programme. New York: United Nations.

Available at www.disaster-info.net/lideres/spanish/mexico/biblio/eng/doc13980.pdf

Kailes, J. I. (2005a). *Disaster services and "special needs": Terms of art or meaningless term?* Lawrence: University of Kansas, Research and Training Center on Independent Living. Available at http://www2.ku.edu/~rrtcpbs/findings/pdfs/SpecialsNeeds.pdf.

Kailes, J. I. (2005b). *Why and how to include people with disabilities in your emergency planning process?* Lawrence: University of Kansas, Research and Training Center on Independent Living.

Kass, N. E. (2001). An ethics framework for public health. *American Journal of Public Health, 91*, 1776–1782.

Kass N. E. (2004). Public health ethics: From foundations and frameworks to justice and global public health. *Journal of Law, Medicine & Ethics, 32*, 232–42.

Kass N. E. (2005). An ethics framework for public health and avian influenza pandemic preparedness. *Yale Journal of Biology and Medicine, 78*, 239–54.

Keystone Center. (2007). *Pandemic influenza vaccine prioritization: Public engagement meetings.* Keystone, CO: Author.

King's Fund. (2004). *Public attitudes to public health.* London: The King's Fund.

Kinlaw, K., Barrett, D. H., & Levine, R. J. (2009). Ethical guidelines in pandemic influenza: Recommendations of the Ethics Subcommittee of the Advisory Committee of the Director, Centers for Disease Control and Prevention. *Disaster Medicine and Public Health Preparedness, 3*(Suppl 2), 1–8.

Knobler, S., Mahmoud, A., Lemon, S., Mack, A., Sivitz, L., & Oberholtzer, K. (Eds.). (2004b). *Learning from SARS: Preparing for the next disease outbreak.* Institute of Medicine, Forum on Microbial Threats, Board on Global Health. Washington, DC: National Academies Press. Available at http://www.nap.edu/catalog/10915/learning-from-sars-preparing-for-the-next-disease-outbreak-workshop.

Knobler, S. L., Mack, A., Mahmoud, A., & Lemon, S. M. (Eds.). (2004a). *The threat of pandemic influenza: Are we ready?* Workshop summary. Institute of Medicine Forum on Microbial Threats, Board on Global Health. Washington, DC: National Academies Press. Available at: http://www.nap.edu/download.php?record_id=11150.

Krimsky, S., & Golding, D. (Eds.). (1992). *Social theories of risk.* Westport, CT: Praeger.

Langewiesche, W. (2002). *American ground: Unbuilding the World Trade Center*. New York: North Point.

Levine, C. (2004). The concept of vulnerability in disaster research. *Journal of Traumatic Stress, 17*, 395–402.

Lukes, S. (2006). Questions about power: Lessons from the Louisiana hurricane. In *Understanding Katrina: Perspectives from the social sciences*. Social Science Research Council. Available at http://understandingkatrina.ssrc.org/Lukes/.

MacIntyre, A. (2007). *After virtue: A study in moral theory* (3rd edition). South Bend, IN: University of Notre Dame Press.

Marmot, M. (2004). *The status syndrome: How social standing affects our health and longevity*. New York: Times Books.

Meslin, E. M., Alyea, J. M., & Helft, P. R. (2007). *Pandemic flu preparedness: Ethical issues and recommendations to the Indiana State Department of Health*. Technical advisory document (TAD-05-07). Indianapolis: Indiana University Center for Bioethics.

Messias, D. K., & Lacy, E. (2007). Katrina-related health concerns of Latino survivors and evacuees. *Journal of Health Care for the Poor and Underserved, 18*, 443–464.

Molotch, H. (2006). Death on the roof: Race and bureaucratic failure. In *Understanding Katrina: Perspectives from the social sciences*. Social Science Research Council. Available at http://understandingkatrina.ssrc.org/Molotch/.

National Council on Disability. (2008). *Saving lives: Including people with disabilities in emergency planning*. Washington, DC: National Press Club.

National Organization on Disability. (2008). *Prepare yourself: Disaster readiness tips for people with disabilities*. Washington, DC: National Organization on Disability.

New York State Workgroup on Ventilator Allocation in an Influenza Pandemic, NYS DOH/NYS Task Force on Life and the Law (2007). *Allocation of ventilators in an influenza pandemic: Planning document*. New York State Department of Health. Available at http://www.health.state.ny.us/diseases/communicable/influenza/pandemic/ventilators/docs/ventilator_guidance.pdf.

Nuffield Council on Bioethics. (2007). *Public health: Ethical issues*. London: Author.

Oliver-Smith, A (2006). Disasters and forced migration in the 21st century. In *Understanding Katrina: Perspectives from the social sciences*. Social Science Research Council. Available at http://understandingkatrina.ssrc.org/Oliver-Smith/.

O'Mathúna, D. P., Gordijn, B., & Clarke, M. (Eds.). (2014). *Disaster bioethics: Normative issues when nothing is normal.* Dordrecht: Springer Press.

Parmet, W. E. (2007). Legal power and legal rights. Isolation and quarantine in the case of drug-resistant tuberculosis. *New England Journal of Medicine, 357*, 433–435.

Pastor, M., Bullard, R. D., Boyce, J. K., Fothergill, A., Morello-Frosch, R., & Wright, B. (2006). *In the wake of the storm: Environment, disaster and race after Katrina.* New York: Russell Sage Foundation.

Paton, D., & Johnston, D. (2006). *Disaster resilience: An integrated approach.* Springfield, IL: Charles C. Thomas.

Pelling, M. (2003). *The vulnerability of cities: Natural disasters and social resilience.* Sterling, VA: Earthscan.

Person, B., Sy, F., Holton, K., Govert, B., Liang, A., & NCID/SARS Community Outreach Team (2004). Fear and stigma: The epidemic within the SARS outbreak. Emerging Infectious Diseases, *10*, 359–363.

Powers, M., & Faden, R. (2006). *Social justice: The moral foundations of public health and health policy.* Oxford: Oxford University Press.

Prehn, A. W., & Vawter, D. E. (2008). *Ethical guidance for rationing scarce health-related resources in a severe influenza pandemic: Literature and plan review.* Minneapolis: Minnesota Center for Health Care Ethics and University of Minnesota Center for Bioethics.

Putnam, R. D. (2000). *Bowling alone.* New York: Simon and Schuster.

Reid, L. (2005). Diminishing returns? Risk and the duty to care in the SARS epidemic. *Bioethics, 19*, 353.

Rosner, D., & Markovitz, G. (2006). *Are we ready? Public health since 9/11.* Berkeley: University of California Press.

Saunders, G. L., & Monet, T. (2007). Eliminating injustice toward disadvantaged populations during an influenza pandemic. *North Carolina Medical Journal, 68*(1), 46–48.

Savitch, H. V. (2008). *Cities in a time of terror: Space, territory, and local resilience.* Armonk, NY: M. E. Sharp.

Scanlon, J. (2006). Two cities, two evacuations: Some thoughts on moving people out. In *Understanding Katrina: Perspectives from the social sciences.* Social Science Research Council. Available at http://understandingkatrina.ssrc.org/Scanlon/.

Scarry, E. (2011). *Thinking in an emergency.* New York: W. W. Norton.

Schafer, W. A., Carroll, J. M., Haynes, S. R., & Abrams, S. (2008). Emergency management planning as collaborative community work. *Journal of Homeland Security and Emergency Management,*

5(1), ISSN (Online) 1547-7355, DOI: 10.2202/1547-7355.1396, March 2008.

Schoch-Spana, M., Franco, C., Nuzzo, J. B., & Usenza, C. (2007). Community engagement: Leadership tool for catastrophic health events. *Biosecurity and Bioterrorism: Biodefense Strategy Practice and Science, 5*, 8–25.

Schön, D. A. (1984). *The reflective practitioner.* New York: Basic Books.

Schön, D. A., & Rein, M. (1997). *Frame reflection: Toward the resolution of intractable policy controversies.* New York: Basic Books.

Selznick, P. (1949/1984). *TVA and the grass roots.* Berkeley: University of California Press.

Sen, A. K. (1983). *Poverty and famines: An essay on entitlement and deprivation.* New York: Oxford University Press.

Silver, N. (2012). *The signal and the noise: Why so many predictions fail—but some don't.* New York: Penguin Press.

Smith, K. E. (2013). *Beyond evidence based policy in public health: The interplay of ideas.* Basingstoke, UK: Palgrave Macmillan.

Solnit, R. (2009). *A paradise built in hell: The extraordinary communities that arise in a disaster.* New York: Viking.

Spence, P. R., Lachlan K. A., & Burke J. M. (2007). Adjusting to uncertainty: Coping strategies among the displaced after Hurricane Katrina. *Sociological Spectrum, 27*, 653–678.

Spence, P. R., Lachlan K. A., & Griffin, D. R. (2007). Crisis communications, race, and natural disasters. *Journal of Black Studies, 37*, 539–554.

Strolovitch, D., Warren, D., & Frymer, P. (2006). Katrina's political roots and divisions: Race, class, and federalism in American politics. In *Understanding Katrina: Perspectives from the social sciences.* Social Science Research Council. Available at http://understandingkatrina.ssrc.org/FrymerStrolovitchWarren/.

Sunstein, C. R. (2007). *Worst-case scenarios.* Cambridge, MA: Harvard University Press.

Sze, J. (2006). Toxic soup redux: Why environmental racism and environmental justice matter after Katrina. In *Understanding Katrina: Perspectives from the social sciences.* Social Science Research Council. Available at http://understandingkatrina.ssrc.org/Sze/.

Thaler, R. H., & Sunstein, C. R. (2008). *Nudge: Improving decisions about health, wealth, and happiness.* New Haven, CT: Yale University Press.

Thomas, J. C., Sage, M., Dillenberg, J., & Guillory, V. J. (2002). A code of ethics for public health. *American Journal of Public Health, 92*, 1057–1059.

Tracy, L. (2007). *Muddy waters: The legacy of Katrina and Rita*. Washington, DC: American Public Health Association.

Trotter, G. (2007). *The ethics of coercion in mass casualty medicine*. Baltimore, MD: Johns Hopkins University Press.

United Nations. (2004). *A more secure world: Our shared responsibility*. Report of the Secretary-General's high-level panel on threats, challenges and change. United Nations. Available at http://www.un.org/en/peacebuilding/pdf/historical/hlp_more_secure_world.pdf.

University of Florida. Cooperative Extension Service. Institute of Food and Agricultural Sciences. (1998). Disaster planning for elderly and disabled populations. In Charles Brown, Carol Magary, and Ami Neiberger (Eds.). *The disaster handbook*. Gainesville: University of Florida. Available at http://disaster.ifas.ufl.edu/chap2fr.htm.

University of Toronto Joint Centre for Bioethics. (2005). *Stand on guard for thee: Ethical considerations in preparedness planning for pandemic influenza*. Toronto: University of Toronto Joint Centre for Bioethics. Available at http://www.jointcentreforbioethics.ca/publications/documents/stand_on_guard.pdf.

Upshur, R. E. (2002). Principles for the justification of public health intervention. *Canadian Journal of Public Health, 93*, 101–103.

US Department of Homeland Security. (2005). *Individuals with disabilities and emergency preparedness (Executive Order 13347). Annual report, July 2005*. Washington, DC: Author. Available at http://www.dhs.gov/xlibrary/assets/CRCL_IWD. E.P_AnnualReport_2005.pdf.

US Department of Justice. (2006). *Making community emergency preparedness and response programs accessible to people with disabilities*. Available at http://www.ada.gov/emergencyprep.htm.

Uscher-Pines, L., Duggan, P. S., Garoon, J. P., Karron, R. A., & Faden, R. R. (2007). Planning for an influenza pandemic: Social justice and disadvantaged groups. *Hastings Center Report, 37*, 32–39.

Vale, L. J., & Campanella, T. J. (2005). *The resilient city: How modern cities recover from disaster*. New York: Oxford University Press.

Vawter, D. E., Garrett, J. E., Gervais, K. G., Prehn, A. W., DeBruin, D. A., Tauer, C. A., . . . Marshall M. F. (2010a). *For the good of us all: Ethically rationing health resources in Minnesota in a severe influenza pandemic*. St. Paul: Minnesota Center for Health Care Ethics and University of Minnesota Center for Bioethics. Available at http://www.health.state.mn.us/divs/idepc/ethics/.

Vawter, D. E., Garrett, J. E., Gervais, K. G., Prehn, A. W., & DeBruin, D. A. (2010b). Dueling ethical frameworks for allocating health resources. *American Journal of Bioethics, 10*(4), 54–56. doi: 10.1080/15265161003632989.

Vawter, D. E., Garrett, J. E., Gervais, K. G., Prehn, A. W., & DeBruin D. A. (2011). Attending to social vulnerability when rationing pandemic resources. *Journal of Clinical Ethics, 22*(1), 42–53. Available at http://www.clinicalethics.com/single_article/na3ecrwzanA.html.

Vawter, D. E., Garrett, J. E., Prehn, A. W., & Gervais, K. G. (2008). Health care workers' willingness to work in a pandemic. *American Journal of Bioethics, 8*(8), 21–23. doi: 10.1080/15265160802318204.

Vawter, D. E., Gervais, K. G., Garrett, J. E., & Pandemic Influenza Ethics Work Group (2007). Allocating pandemic influenza vaccines in Minnesota: Recommendations of the pandemic influenza ethics work group. *Vaccine, 25*(35), 6522–6536.

Verweij, M. (2006). *Project on addressing ethical issues in pandemic influenza planning: Equitable access to therapeutic and prophylactic measures*. Geneva: World Health Organization.

Walker, B., & Salt, D. (2006). *Resilience thinking: Sustaining ecosystems and people in a changing world*. Washington, DC: Island Press.

Walzer, M. (1973). Political action: The problem of dirty hands. *Philosophy and Public Affairs, 2*, 160–180.

Wilkinson, R. G. (1996). *Unhealthy societies: The afflictions of inequality*. London: Routledge.

Wilkinson, R. G., & Pickett, K. (2009). *The spirit level: Why greater equality makes societies stronger*. New York: Bloomsbury.

Williams, A. (1997). Intergenerational equity: An exploration of the "fair innings" argument. *Health Economics, 6*, 117–132.

Wizemann, T., Reeve, M., & Altevogt, B. M. (Rapporteurs). (2013a). *Engaging the public in critical disaster planning and decision making: Workshop summary*. Institute of Medicine Forum on Medical and Public Health Preparedness for Catastrophic Events, Board on Health Sciences Policy. Washington, DC: National Academies Press. Available at http://www.nap.edu/download.php?record_id=18396.

Wizemann, T., Reeve, M., & Altevogt B. M. (Rapporteurs). (2013b). *Preparedness, response, and recovery considerations for children and families: Workshop summary.* Institute of Medicine Forum on Medical and Public Health Preparedness for Catastrophic Events, Board on Health Sciences Policy. Washington, DC: National Academies Press. Available at http://www.nap.edu/download.php?record_id=18550.

World Health Organization. (2007). *Ethical considerations in developing a public health response to pandemic influenza.* Geneva: World Health Organization. Available at http://www.who.int/csr/resources/publications/WHO_CDS_EPR_GIP_2007_2/en/index.html.

World Trade Center Health Panel. (2007). *Addressing the health impacts of 9/11, Report and recommendations to Mayor Michael R. Bloomberg.* New York City Government, Office of the Mayor. Available at http://www.nyc.gov/html/om/pdf/911_health_impacts_report.pdf.

Wray, R., Rivers, J., Whitworth, A., Jupka, K., & Clements, B. (2006). Public perceptions about trust in emergency risk communication: Qualitative research findings. *International Journal of Mass Emergencies and Disasters, 24*, 45–75.

Zack, N. (2009). *Ethics for disaster.* Lanham, MD: Rowman and Littlefield.

2

Justice, Resource Allocation, and Emergency Preparedness

Issues Regarding Stockpiling

NORMAN DANIELS

Overview

Because disease and disability impair normal functioning, they limit the range of opportunities people would otherwise have, given their talents and skills. Therefore, health—or normal functioning—is of special moral importance from the perspective of social justice because it makes a limited but significant contribution to the range of opportunities open to people (Daniels, 1985, 2008). If, as many believe, society has an obligation to promote equality of opportunity, then it has a social obligation to promote population health and to distribute that health equitably. Meeting this obligation requires a just distribution of all the determinants of health, including public health services and personal medical services (Daniels, Kennedy, & Kawachi, 1999, 2000).

Many health needs arise regularly and predictably and must be planned for accordingly. Other population health needs arise less predictably as a result of natural and manmade emergencies. The obligation to protect population health and distribute it fairly should accordingly also govern the approach to emergency preparedness, including the need for stockpiling medical supplies and treatments for a range of health emergencies. These obligations apply in regional emergencies following natural disasters or more localized forms of chemical and radiologic terrorism; they also apply in national or international health emergencies that might follow natural pandemics or some forms of biological terrorism.

What principles, considerations, or procedures should play a role in planning for population health emergencies, including developing stockpiles of medical resources? The traditional emphasis in public health planning is on health maximization strategies—either minimizing the aggregate impact of certain health problems (e.g., lowering mortality rates, maternal mortality rates, or infant mortality rates) or maximizing certain measures of health benefits (e.g., life expectancy to life years or quality-adjusted life years [QALYs] gained or disability adjusted life years [DALYs] saved). More recently, however, the public health movement has paid more attention to promoting equity in health, both at national and international levels (World Health Organization Europe, 2002; World Health Organization Regional Office of Europe, 1999). In a simple maximizing principle or strategy, distributive effects can be comfortably ignored, and public health officials may have a clearer sense about their obligations, although they still face problems arising from uncertainty. When they realize that obligations of justice involve the pursuit of both equity and population health improvement, however, clarity and agreement on goals are harder to reach. People will disagree about how to resolve conflicts among these objectives. This perplexing problem arises in emergency planning as well as in meeting standard health needs. In both contexts, an appeal to principles must be supplemented with reliance on a fair, deliberative process (Daniels & Sabin, 1997).

Planning for emergencies is not itself an emergency situation. Planners should not be tempted into thinking that all nuance or subtlety about ethical obligations can be finessed because they are considering a crisis situation. Proper planning ensures that due care is taken regarding how to meet moral obligations in actual emergencies. In this chapter, I examine more systematically the conflict between maximization and equity, especially as it arises in the context of stockpiling for emergencies. Because the many disagreements that arise about all of these matters are ethical in nature, questions about the legitimacy and fairness of stockpile design and other questions of emergency preparedness will be addressed. To that end, I shall briefly describe the kind of fair, deliberative process that should be used in planning for public health emergencies. The account of fair process provides a framework for thinking about community participation in planning and the proper communication of decisions.

Emergency Preparedness Versus Other Health Needs

A Continuum Versus Exceptionalism

Justice requires that normal functioning be protected in a population and that the health that results be distributed. This is optimally accomplished if there is a just distribution of the social determinants of health (including basic liberties, education, effective political participation, control over life and work, income and wealth) as well as an equitable public health and medical system. Such a system would emphasize health risk reduction, the equitable distribution of risks, and appropriate forms of medical prevention and treatment for chronic and acute health conditions. The relatively predictable prevalence of standard public health and medical needs means that, on a population basis, there is little uncertainty plaguing health planning. At the same time, different health needs compete for scarce resources. As important as health is, it is not the only important good that must be protected or provided, and so resources for health compete with other important social needs and goals. This means the problem of priority setting for resource allocation is pervasive and unavoidable in public health planning, even when problems of uncertainty about population needs are not significant.

Natural disasters, including pandemics, as well as forms of biological, chemical, and radiologic terrorism, add considerable uncertainty to the planning for public health emergencies. The dramatic threat posed by worst-case scenarios for disasters, such as a pandemic on the scale of the 1918 influenza pandemic, may lead some to think that emergency preparedness is not on a continuum with ordinary planning for meeting health needs and that the scale of such threats requires thinking about health needs in an entirely novel way. That is a mistake for two main reasons. First, the best preparation for major emergencies is a properly functioning public health system that makes appropriate allocation of resources for both emergencies and ordinary needs. Second, the considerations involved in thinking about appropriate resource allocation across the range of emergency and ordinary health needs raise common issues that need common solutions. Emergency preparedness "exceptionalism" would be a self-defeating strategy.

Criticism of "biodefense" that has surfaced in response to new budgets and priorities that emerged after the September 11 attacks and the US anthrax threats of October 2001 should be understood in light of these two points about the relationship between emergency preparedness and public health systems. An awareness of the implications of globalization should also be incorporated into the public health system. Biodefense should not be "us" versus "them" but a focus on how "we"—citizens of the world—can address global health issues. That means standard methods and principles for reasonable health planning must be extended to emergency planning rather than abandoned for some new "war" footing.

One of the institutional implications of the argument that emergency preparedness requires good public health system building is that countries with global health budgets are better positioned to think about appropriate resource allocation than are countries with fragmented health systems and multiple budgets with different incentive structures. If emergency preparedness means stockpiling resources that are then not readily available for meeting ordinary health needs, that is better done as a tradeoff within a global budget. Where different budgets address these competing needs in a more fragmented system, unnecessary redundancies or other kinds of inefficiency and inadequacy in decision-making are more likely to be found. Similarly, compliance with restrictions on resources might be easier to achieve if the resource allocation results from a closed budget that puts all people on the same footing; otherwise, compliance is more readily threatened by "gaming of the system" (Daniels, 1986). Specifically, a mixed system with competing budgets and resources might lead to more rampant forms of hoarding and noncompliance with resource restrictions than a system that places competition for resources on a level playing field.

Uncertainty and Planning

In resource allocation decisions for ordinary public health and medical needs, uncertainty plays only a small role at the population level. It is possible to know the prevalence of various health conditions and make fairly accurate estimates of what is needed to meet them during the course of a budget or planning cycle (Murray & Lopez, 1996). An extensive body of actuarial experience is available that allows accurate projections of medical and most public health needs. In contrast, emergency preparedness poses the problem of uncertainty about needs (What exactly will be the outcome of some health emergency at the population level?) and about probabilities (What exactly is the likelihood of a specific emergency arising in a given time period?). Because there is so much uncertainty about both, considerable disagreement arises about appropriate responses.

Since worst-case scenarios are particularly frightening (e.g., major influenza pandemics that might kill millions of people globally and significantly disrupt economies), people who are especially risk averse will want to devote considerable resources to preparing for these events. They might even defend their perspective by suggesting that when the global stakes are as high as these scenarios suggest, an appropriate rule of choice for planning is to minimize worst outcomes. Others will want to put more effort into planning for more frequent and less serious emergencies. They are less inclined to abandon more standard Bayesian rules of choice even without having great confidence in the estimates of either outcomes or probabilities. There is no clear model of rational planning that resolves such disputes about resource allocation in the face of uncertainty. This source of reasonable disagreement about rational choice has similar implications to the reasonable ethical disagreement about tradeoffs between maximization and equity. Both suggest a need for fair process to establish legitimacy for decision-making.

Actually, the two problems may interact. One author has argued that the reservations that planners have about making "social worth" judgments about individuals in medical need in standard, nonemergency contexts may not be appropriate in serious emergency contexts that involve deep threats to the functioning of society and not merely substantial health needs (Arras, 2005). In effect, in planning for worst-case scenarios, health officials may need to modify views about fair treatment and equal respect for persons that should govern standard contexts. In short, if it is rational to plan for extreme scenarios, then ethical restraints may need to be modified as well. This is not to endorse this conclusion but to note that reasonable people may not only disagree about the weight to be given worst-case scenarios in planning, but they also may invoke different or novel ethical considerations in those contexts as well.

Another consideration about uncertainty is that it may seem reasonable to adopt strategies based on poor-quality evidence when few options are available and the stakes are viewed as very high. An illustration is the World Health Organization (WHO) recommendations regarding treatment and prophylactic use of oseltamivir for H5N1 viral infections in humans (Shunemann, Hill, & Kakad, 2007). Despite weak and indirect evidence for the effectiveness of oseltamivir against H5N1 for either treatment or prophylactic purposes (there is only some indirect evidence from animal models for H5N1 and from uses of the drug for seasonal influenza), the high fatality associated with the illness and the absence of other treatment and prophylaxis regimens led to strong recommendations for its use from an international panel of experts. The risk involved in this recommendation is that too much weight is placed on one set of measures for containing a pandemic, at least in the mind of the public and many providers, perhaps to the exclusion of other public health strategies, such as the simple hygiene measures that are a standard first-line of defense and are emphasized as well in pandemic influenza guidelines. A consequence might be that the public becomes overconfident, thinking that adequate steps have been taken to address a potential pandemic because an antiviral drug of questionable effectiveness is recommended and stockpiled. In view of such effects, again disagreement might arise about the strength of the recommendation, given the limited available evidence about the drug's effectiveness.

Maximization in Emergency Preparedness Planning

Maximizing What?

Understanding the rationale for maximization and the targets of maximization is based first on an understanding of utilitarianism. Utilitarianism, one of the most familiar consequentialist ethical frameworks, is a theory with two main parts (Sen & Williams, 1982): one part is a theory about ranking worlds on the "better than" relationship; the other is a consequentialist principle that promotes the aim of producing the best alternative world. For utilitarianism, one world is better than another if it contains more aggregate welfare in it than another, where the principle of aggregation is sum ranking. This is determined by simply adding up all the welfare (conceived of as net pleasure minus pain, or net happiness, or, in more contemporary terms, net satisfaction of preferences) of individuals to arrive at an aggregate welfare for the world containing those individuals. Other welfarist theories might chose a different way of ranking worlds—for example, one world might be better than another if the worst-off group in it is better off than the worst-off group in the other world—but utilitarianism uses this simple principle of sum ranking. The consequentialist normative principle, then, is to aim to produce the world with at least as high a rank as any other.

The goal of utilitarianism is to maximize aggregate welfare (however it is conceived), thus capturing a nonmoral notion of goodness. The theory thus builds on the idea that the right thing to do is to produce a world with the most goodness in it, and this has some intuitive force (Sidgwick, 1907/1966). However, utilitarianism does not simply call for maximizing aggregate health in a population. Maximizing aggregate health might have some tendency to promote goodness in a world, but other things contribute to goodness from a utilitarian perspective and might compete with the straight maximization of health. If, for example, some people contribute more to society, adding more welfare to the world than others, improving their health rather than the health of others would contribute to net welfare more than maximizing health in the aggregate. Keeping working people healthy, for example, produces more indirect benefits from investment in health than keeping retirees or the unemployed healthy, so, following utilitarian thinking, health resources would be allocated where they produce the greatest aggregate welfare, which may not be the same thing as where they produce the greatest aggregate health.

When public health approaches maximize health and ignore other goods that may contribute to welfare, they depart from strict utilitarian principles. Such a departure may be justifiable, but not from a utilitarian perspective. For example, some might argue that emergency preparedness and response (EPR) planners must show equal respect for people and interpret that to mean that they should not make judgments about the social worth or social contribution of individuals when assessing their competing claims for health needs. Rather, they must assess the strength of their claims according to their needs alone. Such a view is a departure from a theory that stresses maximizing aggregate welfare.

The article cited previously (Arras, 2005) argues for equal respect in ordinary situations where the social fabric is not seriously threatened. Where the social fabric is threatened, as in some general health emergencies, health officials may consider the contributions of various people to maintaining the social order and assign priorities accordingly. One form of this argument is that there should be less reluctance to embrace broader utilitarian concerns when the stakes are very high in the aggregate, as they are when the social fabric is so threatened. In effect, the argument states that planners can afford to be concerned about equal respect when the stakes are modest, but when they are very great, they should focus on avoiding great harms.

A critic of this view might counter that the more privileged and powerful people during a time of crisis will always assert their greater social contribution and steer benefits to themselves. The consequence will be that relaxing scruples in time of crisis opens the door to serious errors about real social utility. Even if public health planners focus on avoiding great harms, including threats to the functioning of key social institutions, they are not likely to succeed if they ignore the principle of equal respect. Claims from well-situated people about their societal importance are likely to be confused with more objective assessments of what kinds of tasks are essential to protect.

Maximizing What Measure of Health?

A public health approach that aims at maximizing health in the aggregate, leaving aside other goods—including in times of emergency—must make choices about what measure of health it aims to maximize. Should we save the greatest number of lives? Should we save the greatest number of life years? Or the greatest number of QALYs? Each choice has ethical dimensions that will provoke disagreement.

Considering the choice between maximizing numbers of people saved versus number of life years saved, the latter appears to give priority to saving younger people rather than older ones; the former implies that age should not matter and that life is valuable independently of how much of it has already been experienced. In maximizing lives saved over life years saved, EPR planners might be charged with being insensitive to the greater "need" the young have for more years than the old, or how much worse off they would be dying young than would those who are older, or, as one conception of fair allocation over the life span would have it, that it might be prudent for everyone to favor using scarce resources to maximize life years saved if they did not know how old they are and had to choose. Arguments about fairness pull in both directions, and reasonable people may disagree about them.

In some situations, maximizing lives saved might be preferred, but in reality it proves easier to save more lives in areas of denser population than in more sparsely populated areas. This might lead to concentrating resources in ways that give a much greater chance at being saved to some groups than to others. Maximizing numbers of lives saved is being done at the expense of giving people equal, or even fair, chances at being saved. Some would argue that maximizing numbers of lives saved is a form of favoring "best outcomes" over "fair chances." Others, however, would prefer giving more weight to fair chances than would happen with always favoring best outcomes. Therefore, this particular form of maximization immediately encounters one of the standard distributive problems that has been labeled an "unsolved rationing problem" (Daniels, 1993).

Favoring the maximization of life years saved over lives saved presents another version of the same problem. Here, the best outcome is saving the most life years—that is, favoring the young over those who are older (other things being equal). But this choice means that older people lose all chance—including a fair chance—at any significant benefit so that the young can produce a best outcome. In addition, if maximizing QALYs (or saving DALYs) is favored, planners may readjust what counts as a best outcome, but they still encounter the same distributive problem.

It might be thought that a strategy of saving the most lives would be defensible both on consequentialist and nonconsequentialist grounds because a life saved can be considered a good outcome by a consequentialist, and a principle treating all lives as equally worth saving might seem to be fair to all people since all have claims to be saved. However, a consequentialist might argue for considering the indirect benefits of saving some lives as compared with others, so that more valuable outcomes might result if those lives were saved that contribute more to society. Saving a life is a good, but other goods must be considered as well. Similarly, the nonconsequentialist might complain that some people have stronger claims on being saved than others, perhaps because their dying at a younger age makes them worse off than someone who has lived a considerably longer life. In short, reasonable people will disagree about even the principle some consider most obvious in emergency situations, namely, a principle calling for saving the most lives.

Division of Labor: An Argument for Maximization?

Each choice of what measure of health to maximize produces some version of broader concerns about fairness in the distribution of health benefits. Still, there is some plausibility to thinking that the responsibility of people dedicated to protecting the population's health, including in emergencies, should be concerned with maximizing some measure of health. This is plausible because of the efficiency that results from a proper division of effort or responsibility. If those in public health are charged with maximizing health, they are likely to produce more health than if they are charged with more complex judgments about how to trade health against other goods. Fairness across sectors or spheres, then, becomes a problem for some broader social agency—a democratic political process, perhaps—that is responsible for arriving at an overall fair social policy. But experts within each sphere should be charged with the task of doing what they know how to do best, namely, maximizing the good that sphere is charged with producing. One possible implication of that argument is that public health agencies should pick a measure of health and then aim to maximize it and not be troubled by the nuanced concerns about fairness. Unfortunately, the ethical disagreements noted here would mean that such a strategy would be challenged and would raise questions about the legitimacy of a strategy that deliberately ignored concerns about fairness.

Does Helping Worst-Off Lead to Maximizing Aggregate Health?

A further, traditional support for adopting a maximizing strategy is the hope, often expressed by proponents of public health, that the most successful strategy for promoting aggregate health is to improve the health of those with worse health. This group can make the biggest gains and thus contribute the most to maximizing population health in the aggregate. In eradication efforts for some infectious diseases, substantial gains in measures of aggregate health have resulted from efforts to help the poor with endemic conditions.

Although this may hold for some public health programs, it is not in general true. Worst-off groups may be very inefficient converters of resources into health compared with somewhat better-off groups, so one cannot assume that health maximization and giving priority to those worst off pull in the same direction in general. Indeed, various social science studies have found that many people are willing to trade maximization of aggregate health for making more modest gains that improve those who are worst off. In short, health maximization does not follow, at least in general, from targeting the worst-off parts of the population.

Maximization Versus Equity: The Case of Stockpiling

An illustration of how reasonable disagreement arises about key choices in emergency planning is the development of stockpiles of key medical resources. I believe there is a lack of consensus on fine-grained principles that could resolve some disputes about these choices in the goals and design of a stockpile. In the absence of such a consensus, a plan will have legitimacy and be perceived as fair only if it is developed in a way that ensures accountability for its reasonableness. The issues of legitimacy concern more than simply who decides: legal authority, and perhaps moral authority, for decision-making may be clear, but how decisions are made also affects legitimacy. In the following paragraphs, key choice points about stockpiling will be discussed. I will describe the conditions that a fair deliberative process must meet if it is to establish the legitimacy and fairness of the choices made.

Stockpiling and Public Goods Versus the Concept of "Shared Responsibility"

A policy debate that cuts across many of the specific issues regarding stockpiling is that of "shared responsibility." Shared responsibility is the claim that the federal government does not have sole responsibility for providing protection to people in the context of medical emergencies, such as an influenza pandemic. Rather, since benefits accrue to many people and many institutions, responsibility for providing those benefits can be divided across federal, state, and local levels, both public and private. Ultimately, shared responsibility could devolve to individuals as well, who might, for example, have the responsibility to acquire and fill a prescription for prophylaxis or treatment use of an antiviral drug.

A basic consideration of social justice is the role of the government in providing for public goods. In contrast to liberal egalitarian views that assign to the government broad obligations to protect the well-being of groups and individuals, even theories of justice that assign a modest role to the government generally agree that it has a special obligation to protect the provision of public goods. Providing security against infection in the context of pandemics is one such obligation; police powers of quarantine derive from this obligation to provide security, not only from external aggression but also from infectious disease as well. If individuals can be prevented from becoming infected, they will not infect others. Being kept free from infection is thus not just a good for the individual but also affects the security of others. If individuals are left to protect themselves, and some fail to act responsibly or cannot protect themselves because of limits on their resources, this then exposes third parties to substantial harms. It is this feature of protection from infectious disease that necessitates assigning primary responsibility to society—to government—for providing the public good of health protection in the context of infectious disease.

Some specific obligations might be assigned to specific institutions in order to ensure the effective provision of the public good. Such obligations could fall to various federal, tribal, state, and local public agencies, as well as to various private organizations. That assignment of responsibility would require the force of law or regulation, and it would have to be backed up with sanctions and strong forms of accountability. It could not be left to the private or voluntary assumption of "responsibility" because people may find excuses for why other things take priority over this responsibility. If, for example, certain private corporations failed to purchase and provide oseltamivir prophylaxis to their employees, they might pay the private penalty of losing part of their workforce. Those employees are then likely to infect others as a result of their not being "responsibly" protected. These externalized harms point to the need for stronger assurance that the public good of protection is provided. The state cannot escape its obligation to provide a public good through attempting to pass on assumed responsibilities. However, with the appropriate legal and regulatory framework, the obligation can devolve to appropriately accountable entities, both public and private.

Assigning those obligations, however, will raise important issues of justice. If private entities are required to assume such obligations, then it is fair to expect them to be able to meet those obligations. For example, small-scale private purchases of antiviral drugs are likely to be much more costly than large-scale purchases at government rates. Individuals, groups, or institutions without the resources to meet those obligations cannot be required to do so without appropriate redistribution of resources. Blanket appeals to individual, corporate, or even community responsibility are not a substitute for careful assessment of the fairness of assigning obligations to those entities, given their actual capabilities to meet the obligations.

In short, the concept of "shared responsibility" seems to fit more naturally with the provision of individual goods, not public goods. Where public goods, like protection of a public against infection, are involved, the more appropriate concept from the perspective of justice is "obligation," not the weaker notion of responsibility; and where the obligations are to be shared, there must be adequate attention paid to the fairness of the distribution of the obligations. Appealing to a notion of shared obligations to provide a public good does not avoid questions about distributive justice; it simply raises those questions in another form. If the issue is how to divide the burden of paying for protection against a pandemic, for example, then society cannot distribute obligations to pay for parts of that burden without being sure it is just or fair to do so. The danger of the language of "shared responsibility" is that it may smuggle into the "sharing" a notion of a different kind of good (i.e., a private good that one can choose to have or not have, when in fact the decision not to have the good imposes risks on third parties that are not consented to and are arguably unjust).

This does not constitute an argument against federalism, which is thought of as a division of obligation between federal and state governments. Nevertheless, one caution does apply to the issue of federalism; that is, there are externalities to state-level actions that may require strong forms of federal regulation. If one state fails to purchase drugs needed for treatment, for example, and symptomatic residents infect other people, the consequences extend beyond state boundaries. Indeed, some metropolitan areas straddle state lines, and ongoing interstate commerce, including the movement of workers, means that treatment and containment efforts must be coordinated across state lines. Where there is a risk of state-level failure to contribute to the provision of the public good of protection against infection, there must be stronger federal control. This does not mean that obligations cannot devolve onto states for purchase of some medical supplies, but only that there must be strong forms of accountability for federalist divisions of obligation. Here, too, "responsibility" may be too weak a term.

Goals or Objectives of Stockpiling for Pandemics

The goals or objectives of stockpiling medical resources for a pandemic are often coupled with specific prioritization strategies for their use. Thus, if a vaccine or antiviral drug were in short supply, it might best be used selectively to try to contain an outbreak; if it is plentiful, it might best be used to protect everyone. If it is being used to protect everyone, the remaining prioritization questions have to do with the sequence of the administration or distribution effort, and such choices may involve different degrees of risk for different groups. This combination of goal selection and prioritization issues can be used to illustrate how ethical disagreement can surround many stockpiling choices and, ultimately, to argue the need for fair process. Although a national stockpile may seem to avoid the prioritization issues because states may be responsible for determining how to prioritize the use of resources released from a national stockpile, it is nevertheless important to understand the distributive issues that arise as a result of the combination of resource scarcity and prioritization decisions, regardless of how authority for making them is currently divided.

A preliminary point that cuts across these cases is that the scarcity of a resource in a stockpile may result from quite different factors. It might result from an initial decision that underestimates what the needs will be, from a budget limitation, or from problems in the market for the drug or device (i.e., too few producers or too little being produced). Sometimes, the decision that creates the scarcity may be criticized on ethical grounds; sometimes the scarcity is not itself the result of bad decisions, but the prioritization decisions that are then made because of the scarcity may themselves be subject to criticism.

Vaccines and Their Uses

To illustrate ethical disagreements that might focus on vaccine use, I present hypothetical cases and distinguish among them. First, suppose that a vaccine for a potentially pandemic avian influenza is available early in an outbreak. If it is available in quantities capable of protecting the whole population, the only prioritization issues concern staging of the mass vaccination campaign. Such prioritization questions may involve some additional risks to those who are among the last groups to be vaccinated. Suppose, for example, urban populations were to be vaccinated first, in part because the risk of early outbreak was estimated to be higher in more densely populated areas. Still, given population mobility, including workers commuting to cities and others visiting or shopping there, some risk remains to nonurban populations that is ignored by the prioritization. People in the areas where immunization campaigns are delayed could argue that they are being denied a chance at a substantial benefit (early protection) because a best outcome (i.e., preventing the most cases) is achievable by giving priority to urban populations.

Put in this form, their complaint would be a version of the classic "best outcomes versus fair chances" distributive problem. The nonurban people who are at some risk, even if at less risk than urbanites, can complain that they are being asked to forgo all chances at early protection so that others, at admittedly higher risk, can obtain a better outcome. Reasonable people might then disagree about how much weight or priority to give best outcomes versus giving more people a fair chance at some benefit. Even if they agree that always favoring best outcomes is unfair to those with less than best outcomes, they may not agree on how to weigh the two considerations: fair chances at some benefit versus better outcomes. Some propose a proportional "lottery" that takes both factors into account, although just how the proportions are established remains a point of controversy (Brock, 1988; Kamm, 1993).

The problem may be characterized in another way. The urban population has a higher risk of early infection. In this regard, it is "worst off" than the lower risk nonurban population. The prioritization strategy might then seem to be a case of giving priority to those who are worst off, which is an equity consideration favored by many. However, giving the worst off complete priority, regardless of the benefits forgone by others, seems unacceptable to many, but giving no priority to the worst off is also unacceptable to many. But how much priority should we give them? (I have previously labeled this unsolved problem the "priorities problem" [Daniels, 1993].) To illustrate, the objection from the nonurban population might be recast as follows: giving complete priority to the urban population and ignoring providing any early protection to those at (admittedly) lower risk, but still at some risk, is a case of giving too much priority to those who are worst off. Perhaps it is possible to identify the subgroups of the nonurban population at comparable risk to subgroups of the urban population and to extend as much protection to them. Reasonable people will disagree about how to weigh the alternative strategies. Even if the example is changed to suggest that the vaccine is not in abundant supply, but is in limited supply, this brings up variations on the same distributive problems.

Antiviral Treatment and Prophylaxis

Other distributive problems arise in the context of stockpiling as well, and these may be better illustrated by the example of antiviral drugs. Suppose there is a supply of antiviral drugs, such as oseltamivir, which can be used for treatment, but the drug is not in adequate supply to treat everyone who could potentially benefit from it. Suppose, for example, it is less effective for persons with more advanced symptoms than it is for those with recent exposure who could take it either as treatment (with early symptoms) or as prophylaxis (if not yet symptomatic). Suppose, however, that those with the more serious cases sometimes benefit from treatment, perhaps avoiding more serious morbidity or even death, and suppose further that this benefit is produced only at higher dosages, thus decreasing the benefit that might be given to others with less serious disease or as prophylaxis.

Again, there are two ways to describe this kind of example. If health officials give the drug to those with serious illness, despite its lesser effectiveness, they are giving greater priority to those already worse off. Those who would then have to forgo earlier treatment or prophylaxis could complain that too much priority has been given to those who are worse off, and health officials have ignored important claims that others at risk have on resources. If, however, they favor "best outcomes" and then reserve the drug for use by those who will get more benefit from it, then the already seriously ill persons who give up any chance at benefit can complain that they are being sacrificed to the better outcomes of others. It is not fair that they give up all chance at any (significant) benefit so that others may benefit more.

Either way the distributive problem is described, it involves ethical disagreement. Moreover, reasonable people will take different positions on these disagreements. There is no way simply to dismiss one or another position as irrational or based on irrelevant considerations.

These "unsolved rationing problems" hardly exhaust the reasonable ethical disagreements encountered in choices about how to use stockpiled resources. One further general problem focuses on the question of whether certain groups, identified by their roles or functions, should be given priority in access to treatment or preventive protections. There is probably widespread support, for example, for giving priority to those who are expected to face exceptional risks from contact with people who can infect others. Many people would support giving priority access to preventive measures to the first responders of various kinds (e.g., emergency medical technicians and fire and police personnel) and health care workers (e.g., physicians, nurses, or other technicians), who are at higher risk but whose expertise is necessary to providing care during a pandemic. However, despite the support many give to such a prioritization, others worry that it violates basic concerns about showing equal respect for all persons, despite their social contribution. The so-called "God" committee that once functioned at a Seattle hospital has long been held up as an example of what should not be done in medical settings. The committee made life-and-death choices about access to renal dialysis early in the development of that technology that were based on questionable criteria about social worth (stable job and family, church attendance) (Levine, 2009). The complaint against singling out people for special medical priority because of their social role or contribution is that it risks importing questionable social worth judgments into a setting where medical need should be the sole criterion for access to services. If that is the criterion, then (or so the argument goes) persons should be shown equal respect.

Sometimes it is argued that a principle of reciprocity implies that special priority should be given to those who are expected to take special risks. The principle of reciprocity, in this view, allows people to favor giving priority to some people over others without violating their concern for equal respect. They are not judging the social worth of health care personnel (for example) but acknowledging the special burden they face by offering them compensatory protection. Note that this argument from reciprocity would not give comparable priority to those performing other essential tasks but who are not at extra risk and who are not expected to act in the face of those extra risks. A further problem with the appeal to the principle of reciprocity in this way is that, as stated, it balances risk taking with risk reduction. In addition, some might think a principle of reciprocity can be applied more broadly and can balance other considerations—perhaps providing rewards for other social contributions. If so, the principle both opens the door to challenging the concern for equal respect and also to a much broader justification of other priorities. Any socially essential task might be thought worthy of reciprocity in the form of special protection. The problem here is general: there is not a clear idea of the scope of the principle being invoked as a principle of reciprocity, and so reasonable people will have disagreements about what it implies. Far from resolving the disagreement referred to earlier, it may add to it.

Ventilators

The stockpiling of ventilators to meet a "surge" in need during a pandemic raises further ethical issues. Some of these issues arise at the federal level, but others may primarily be a matter for states to address, given that states will have to formulate policies for the use of resources released to them from a national stockpile.

The first key ethical issue that arises at the federal level is how large a stockpile of respirators to create. Ventilators, unlike vaccines or antiviral drugs, cannot be stockpiled in quantities adequate to meet the estimated need for them in pandemic worst-case scenarios. The cost for such stockpiling would simply be too great; arguably, the gap in production capacity for ventilators adds a market-based reason for thinking there is no possibility of meeting the needs of a worst-case scenario. But even if stockpiling for a worst-case scenario is not possible, people will disagree about what level of investment is reasonable, and there is no principled way to determine that level. Any budget constraint can seem arbitrary, given that lives may be lost if the stockpile is smaller than it need be. Yet variations in aversion to risk may be one of the key factors shaping people's willingness to invest in stockpiled ventilators.

A second ethical issue at the federal level concerns the judgment about how many ventilators to release to various states as an epidemic unfolds. Giving too many ventilators to states with early outbreaks will be unfair to states that face later outbreaks, but withholding ventilators from those already in need because others may come to need them elsewhere will be challenged by those who need them early. Some people will definitely die because the ventilators are not distributed to some areas, whereas there is only a risk that others will die elsewhere later in the epidemic. If there is a high likelihood that the epidemic will spread, withholding of ventilators will seem geographically more equitable than if the spread is less certain. This, too, is an issue on which reasonable people will disagree and for which there is no principled way to arrive at consensus about a fair distribution.

At the state level, where the supply of ventilators does not meet the need, ethical issues will arise about how to ration their use (New York State Workgroup on Ventilator Allocation in an Influenza Pandemic, 2007). A standard triage procedure would reserve their use for those most likely to survive if they are given ventilators and to exclude those most likely to survive without them or to die with them. Of course, making this judgment is difficult. It is especially difficult if a new patient is more likely to survive if given a ventilator than someone already on it. Switching in such cases may be the strategy that would save the most lives, but it also means abandoning a patient already in treatment, and many health care professionals would find that ethically unacceptable. Even if people agree that switching is acceptable under some conditions, they may disagree about the details of the conditions that make it justifiable.

At both the federal and state levels, then, ethical disagreement will occur among reasonable people who face choices about ventilator stockpiling and uses. Consensus on principles that can resolve these disagreements is lacking. In many contexts of justice, where there is a lack agreement on principles that can resolve a dispute, planners must rely on a fair process and accept the outcome of that process as fair. I discuss this reliance on procedural justice in emergency preparedness further in the following section.

Private Stockpiling

Private stockpiling, if appropriately encouraged and regulated under the right conditions, could supplement public stockpiling in a way that is not unfair and might be efficient. However, if the private stockpiling is done in ways that compete with public stockpiles, it can produce an inefficient and unfair means of dealing with emergency situations. Just what measures should then be taken to address the private hoarding depends on the effect of both the hoarding and efforts to curtail it.

Worries about private stockpiling or hoarding arose in the context of early discussions of an avian influenza pandemic and shortages of oseltamivir. As an example, a prominent physician e-mailed all his friends at the height of the scare about human H5N1 infections during 2007, recommending that they secure supplies of oseltamivir for their families. Obviously, if wealthier, better connected people have a significant impact on a short supply, the chances of stockpiling it for fairer forms of distribution will be undercut. In addition, such stockpiling at retail prices is inefficient. Arguably, it is ineffective as well, since there will be so little clarity about how to use the drug (and no evidence of its effectiveness).

Since 2007, as plans for a national stockpile have advanced and a surge in production has been accomplished, there is less concern about the adequacy of supply of oseltamivir, although federal supplies remain limited because of funding limits, and prophylactic use of federal supplies is not recommended. In the context of a surge in infections and media attention, however, the interest in private stockpiling, temporarily abated, may reemerge. Some of that interest would be based on the public perception, after Hurricane Katrina, that American management of emergencies leaves something to be desired. People may fear that public preparedness cannot be relied upon. In that context, even assuming a national stockpile has been constructed that is adequate to meet the needs for influenza treatment and prophylaxis, some parts of the population will prefer to depend on their own initiative and resources. Under these circumstances, it would be unwise to intervene, since the private initiatives, however inefficient, are unlikely to affect public measures.

Where public preparedness is inadequate, however, private hoarding could pose a significant threat to public initiatives to remedy the situation. Still, if it is unclear that public measures can be significantly improved, stopping the private measures may prevent some unfairness but do so at the expense of denying people the only measures open to them to preserve themselves. The lesson from this is that appropriate, timely emergency preparedness measures are the best protection against widespread private hoarding.

The Need for Fair, Deliberative Process (Accountability for Reasonableness) in Emergency Preparedness Decisions

Legitimacy and Fairness Problems

The fact of life about resource allocation decisions, including those in emergency preparedness contexts, such as stockpiling, is that there are winners and losers. With winners and losers come disagreement and conflict. The conflict in these contexts, however, is not only about competing interests. Reasonable people will often disagree about how to weigh the values that generally compete in these contexts. I have illustrated this point in several ways. There are reasonable disagreements about how to address choices made under uncertainty, about how much priority to give to those who are worst off, about how to weigh the importance of aiming at best outcomes versus giving people a fair chance at some benefit, and about how much to weigh saving more lives against professional obligations not to abandon patients who can benefit from further treatment. These are all value questions, not technical ones. They unavoidably push toward deliberation aimed at morally and politically acceptable, or legitimate, solutions.

Where fundamental issues of well-being are the subject of such moral controversy, decision-makers aspiring to legitimacy must wear a mantle of moral authority. Under what conditions that moral authority is properly accepted as legitimate by those who are affected by the decisions will be referred to as the *legitimacy problem* (Daniels & Sabin 1997, 2002).

The legitimacy problem might seem less difficult, or perhaps no problem at all, if moral authority were easily exercised in the following sense: anyone could check to see if decision-makers make choices that conform with moral principles or reasons on which there is prior consensus. In effect, the public might care less about the conditions establishing legitimacy if the fairness problem had a straightforward, principled solution so that it was clear to all what outcomes counted as fair.

Unfortunately, there is no consensus on such principles and so no simple solution to the fairness problem. Instead, as the examples discussed earlier suggest, there is ongoing controversy surrounding competing values. Without a foreseeable consensus on such principles, EPR planners must find a fair process whose outcomes can be accepted as just or fair. The process must be fair to all who participate in it and who are affected by it; obvious sources of bias or conflict of interest must be removed. Attention must be paid to the voice—the values and interests—of different stakeholders. This is a classic appeal to pure procedural justice (Rawls, 1971), in which we rely on fair process to arrive at a fair outcome in the absence of prior agreement on the criteria or principles governing a fair outcome. This fair process—*accountability for reasonableness*—provides a way to resolve disputes about allocation that are not addressed by more general principles of justice on which people may agree.

Accountability for Reasonableness

Four general conditions ensure accountability for reasonableness. If met, they should, over time, lead members of the public to respect public agency decision-making for its fairness and legitimacy. Although these conditions were originally developed as a general characterization of fair process in health care resource allocation generally, they will be restated here so they focus on the kinds of decisions that must be made in emergency preparedness contexts, for example, in decision-making about the goals and design of a national medical stockpile. The main features of the process are in accord with requirements of public administrative law, so these conditions should readily be met in public agency decision-making. At the same time, the rationale for them provides further grounds for public communication about these decisions.

1. *Publicity condition*: Decisions regarding the goals and means for achieving them, including decisions about priorities in access to resources, as well as the rationales for them must be publicly accessible.

2. *Relevance condition*: These rationales must rest on evidence, reasons, and principles that all fair-minded parties affected by the decisions—managers, clinicians, patients and the public in general—can agree are relevant to deciding how to meet the emergency medical needs of a population under necessary resource constraints. ("Fair-minded parties" are considered people who seek grounds for their decisions that they can mutually justify to each other.)
3. *Revisability condition*: There is a mechanism for challenge and dispute resolution regarding decisions, including the opportunity for revising decisions in light of further evidence or arguments.
4. *Enforcement condition*: There is public regulation of the process to ensure that conditions 1–3 are met.

These four conditions ensure that what might otherwise be largely behind-the-scenes public agency deliberations become a larger, public, ultimately democratic deliberation about using limited resources to protect fairly the health of a population in emergency conditions. The four conditions set the stage for a process of interactive education among all parties, built on accountability. In this way, they provide a foundation for thinking about public communication and education about emergency preparedness and the various obligations and responsibilities that result.

Because emergency preparedness is a context in which resources are clearly limited and priorities have to be set about their use and the criteria that should govern that use, the value of developing a culture of openness about rationales must be recognized. Such openness must take hold against a background in which the US public—and the politicians and health system managers who respond to that public—has little understanding of the need for setting limits or priorities in standard medical contexts. Perhaps the public would be more open to limits in emergencies, but if it has been educated to resist all limits, emergency situations would be more difficult to manage fairly. To change that culture in the long run requires a concerted effort at education, both outside and inside the institutions that deliver care. That education begins with openness about the reasons for the decisions that public or private health providers and insurers make. Over time, this process enables a more focused public deliberation that involves broader democratic institutions. But whether or not the stage is set in this way, it is crucial that decisions made about emergency preparedness engage the public in an open and transparent way.

The publicity condition provides a public record of the ethical commitments to which the agency officials responsible for emergencies adhere in making these kinds of decisions. In effect, the decisions form a kind of case law record, complete with rationales for why decisions are being made. Arguably, this feature improves fairness in decision-making because it provides a basis for judging the coherence and consistency of decisions about emergency preparedness made over time. It gives those affected by decisions, often when they have no real choice to seek alternatives, a way of knowing why they face the restrictions they do. The publicity condition thus satisfies what many believe is a fundamental requirement of justice: the grounds for decisions that fundamentally affect a society's well-being must be publicly available to that society.

The relevance condition imposes important constraints on the kinds of reasons that should play a role in rationales for decisions about goals and priorities. Ideally, it narrows the range of disagreement. The basic idea is that parties pooling resources to face an emergency pursue a common goal or common good. They enter into a plan that aims to meet their diverse needs under necessary resource constraints on terms they can justify to each other. A fair-minded person can be considered someone who believes decisions should be made on grounds that people can justify to each other. Because hard choices will have to be made about how to meet those needs fairly, the grounds for those decisions must be ones that fair-minded persons can agree are relevant to that kind of decision.

Involving various stakeholders in deliberation is one way to secure broader agreement about what count as relevant reasons. Such "buy-in" is important in generating a sense of legitimacy and fairness. However, the main mechanism for improving legitimacy through stakeholder involvement is not an appeal to a form of grassroots democracy. Most stakeholders who can be involved in the deliberation, whether through open hearings, participation in the whole process, or public comment on elements of the process, are not elected representatives who can claim democratic credentials. Because they are not representatives who through a selection process are held accountable to their constituents, their participation should not be seen as making the deliberation "more democratic." Nor do such consumers act as proxy consenters on behalf of other consumers. Instead, they add to the breadth of considerations taken up in the deliberation and, through their effectiveness in representing specific views or considerations, improve the quality of argument. Stakeholder participation is given meaning and direction and a connection to the problem of legitimacy if its goal is to improve accountability for reasonableness. It can do this by enhancing the deliberative process, reassuring various stakeholders their arguments are addressed, broadening perspectives on what counts as relevant reasons, and ensuring the transparency the process requires. At the same time, stakeholders risk distorting deliberation by becoming lobbyists for vested interests. There are both benefits and risks to the broad inclusion of stakeholders in deliberative processes, but the belief is that the benefits significantly outweigh the risks.

Even if it narrows the range of disagreement, the relevance condition obviously does not mean that all parties will agree with the specific decisions made. Parties may agree that reasons are relevant but still give different weight or importance to them. As long as fair-minded parties who make the decision and are affected by it can accept that the grounds for it are relevant, however, then even those who do not like or agree with its specific outcome cannot complain that it is unreasonable. This perceived fairness of the process and its outcomes may act as some barrier against self-protective behavior by those who seek ways around limits set in emergencies, but it would be foolish to think that the barrier makes the result secure against various forms of gaming and cheating. Desperate people will behave in desperate ways, but public perception that people are not being treated unfairly will be key to sustaining support for priorities established in an emergency plan.

Fair-minded people will accept many kinds of evidence and reasons as relevant to emergency decisions. These include scientific evidence about effectiveness and safety. In this regard, as noted earlier, it becomes important to be open about the level of evidence about efficacy that pertains to vaccines and antiviral drugs, both for treatment and prophylaxis. It is also important to be open to new evidence and arguments and to revise components of preparedness, including decisions about stockpiling, as new evidence becomes relevant.

What may be hardest for stakeholders to grasp are budget restrictions that are themselves not justified. Here, there is a cultural conflict between the behavior of managers in public agencies, where traditionally budget decisions are not defended with public rationales, and the strong form of openness demanded by accountability for reasonableness.

Accountability for reasonableness adopts a middle path between the poles of "make everything explicit ahead of time" and "let experts muddle through behind the scenes." The middle path takes the best features from both positions. Like those who advocate explicitness as a condition of fairness, accountability for reasonableness adopts a strong publicity condition. But what is made public need not be a set of principles agreed upon ahead of time; rather, it may be the result of deliberation by experts and other stakeholders about the strongest reasons and arguments supporting a conclusion. Like those who advocate "muddling through" implicitly, accountability for reasonableness draws on the insights that come from examining situations carefully in light of all the evidence.

Conclusion

Emergency preparedness raises many of the same questions of distributive fairness that are raised in other contexts in which resource allocation decisions for health are made. In many of these questions, reasonable people will disagree about how to reconcile concerns about maximizing some measure of aggregate health—including numbers of lives saved in emergency contexts—with concerns about distributing that health fairly. Because consensus is lacking on principles that can resolve those disagreements, EPR planners need to engage in a fair deliberative process to achieve outcomes that are perceived as fair and legitimate. This chapter describes four central conditions that are necessary, if not sufficient, for achieving fairness in such a process. These conditions are compatible with requirements of administrative law and set the stage for appropriate forms of communication with the public about emergency preparedness.

References

Arras, J. D. (2005). Rationing vaccine during an avian influenza pandemic: Why it won't be easy. *Yale Journal of Biology and Medicine, 78*, 287–300.

Brock, D. (1988). Ethical issues in recipient selection for organ transplantation. In Matheiu D. (Ed.), *Organ substitution technology: Ethical, legal and public policy issues*. Boulder, CO: Westview Press, 86–99.

Daniels, N. (1985). *Just health care*. New York: Cambridge University Press.

Daniels, N. (1986). Why saying no to patients in the United States is so hard: Cost containment, justice, and provider autonomy. *New England Journal of Medicine, 314*, 1381–1383.

Daniels, N. (1993). Rationing fairly: Programmatic considerations. *Bioethics, 7*, 224–233.

Daniels, N. (2008). *Just health: Meeting health needs fairly*. New York: Cambridge University Press.

Daniels, N., Kennedy, B., & Kawachi, I. (1999). Why justice is good for our health: The social determinants of health inequalities. *Daedalus, 128*, 215–251.

Daniels, N., Kennedy, B., & Kawachi, I. (2000). *Is inequality bad for our health?* Boston: Beacon Press.

Daniels, N., & Sabin, J. E. (1997). Limits to health care: Fair procedures, democratic deliberation, and the legitimacy problem for insurers. *Philosophy and Public Affairs, 26*, 303–350.

Daniels, N., & Sabin, J. E. (2002). *Setting limits fairly: Can we learn to share medical resources*? New York: Oxford University Press.

Kamm, F. (1993). *Morality, mortality: Death and whom to save from it*, Volume 1. Oxford: Oxford University Press.

Levine, C. (2009). *The Seattle God committee: a cautionary tale*. Health Affairs Blog, November 30. Available at http://healthaffairs.org/blog/2009/11/30/the-seattle-god-committee-a-cautionary-tale/

Murray, C. J. L., & Lopez, A. D. (1996). *The global burden of disease*. Geneva: World Health Organization.

New York State Workgroup on Ventilator Allocation in an Influenza Pandemic. (2007). *Allocation of ventilators in an influenza pandemic: Planning document*. New York State Department of Health/New York State Task Force on Life and the Law. Available at http://www.health.state.ny.us/diseases/communicable/influenza/pandemic/ventilators/docs/ventilator_guidance.pdf.

Rawls, J. (1971). *A theory of justice*. Cambridge, MA: Harvard University Press.

Sen, A., & Williams, B. (1982). *Utilitarianism and beyond*. Cambridge: Cambridge University Press.

Shunemann, H. J., Hill, S. R., & Kakad, M. (2007). WHO rapid advice guidelines for pharmacological management of sporadic human infection with avian influenza A (H5N1) virus. *Lancet Infectious Diseases*, 7, 21–31.

Sidgwick, H. (1907/1966). *The methods of ethics* (7th edition). New York: Dover.

World Health Organization Europe. (2002). *The European health report 2002*. Copenhagen: WHO Regional Office for Europe. WHO Regional Publications, European Series, No. 97. Available at http://www.euro.who.int/document/E76907.pdf.

World Health Organization Regional Office for Europe. (1999). *Health 21: The health for all policy framework for the WHO European Region*. Copenhagen: WHO Regional Office for Europe.

3

Vulnerable Populations in the Context of Public Health Emergency Preparedness Planning and Response

MADISON POWERS

Introduction

Theories of social justice differ in their fundamental theoretical commitments and their practical implications, but almost all but the most radically individualist of moral and political theories contain in their framework the idea that there are some prima facie individual and societal obligations to prevent or mitigate harm to others, at least when the cost of doing so is not unreasonable (Pogge, 2002). Perhaps even wider agreement exists regarding the obligation to prevent or mitigate harm to persons who are especially vulnerable to harms or injuries (Gostin & Powers, 2006).

Whether such obligations rest primarily with governments, particular individuals in social and professional roles, or nongovernmental organizations, most social justice theories agree also on some of the moral obligations of that role. To the extent that a central authority takes on the task on behalf of society, it must conduct itself according to principles of fair regard for the well-being and harm prevention of all its citizens in ways that recognize and respond to the actual vulnerabilities of some segments of the population (Daniels, 1993). More specifically, one concern of justice is to ensure fair distribution, not only of social benefits and opportunities, but also of burdens and risks.

Subpopulations who are at increased risk of preventable harms are due added consideration in the design and implementation of social policies that deal with the impact of a natural disaster, pandemic, or human made emergency. These populations are also due added attention in execution of plans for disaster response. Surveys of disaster-related planning and guidance documents around the world reveal that public health authorities differ considerably in those they identify as especially vulnerable, as well as in the specificity of their plans to address the special needs of the vulnerable. Despite this, the special focus of justice on vulnerable populations has risen to the top of the agenda in many disaster preparedness planning circles (Bellagio Group, 2007*a*, 2007*b*; Uscher-Pines, Duggan, Garoon, Karron, & Faden, 2007).

This chapter examines four major issues. The first section focuses on the relevant notions of vulnerability and the related conceptions of societal duties toward vulnerable populations. Following that is a discussion on what those duties might involve in the way of practical decision and implementation, the relative stringency or priority of duties toward vulnerable populations, and how one might decide what to do when moral duties conflict. The third issue concerns the obligations to gather information, plan for, prevent, or mitigate harm from a disaster, and whether and to what extent these obligations differ in their priority and moral importance. Finally, we consider whether there are significant moral differences associated with different triggering events, such as natural disasters, terrorism, or pandemics.

Conceptions and Attributes of Vulnerability

Types of Loss

All living things are vulnerable to physical injury, disease, and death. Moreover, all sentient beings are vulnerable to pain and suffering. All creatures with any significant degree of complex mental activity are, in addition, subject to the prospect of psychological harms associated with the anticipation or experience of other kinds of losses. For example, fear, anxiety, regret, guilt, shame, grief, confusion, or hopelessness might accompany the experience or anticipation of loss of life, health, economic security, possessions, loved ones, physical security, peace of mind, shelter, sense of place, or the expectations of ordinary life following a disaster. Public health policy planners must be attuned to vulnerabilities to losses of distinct kinds inasmuch as vulnerability must always be understood as some added or special risk for experiencing losses of a specific kind.

Moreover, vulnerabilities to losses of one kind rarely exist in a vacuum or apart from a constellation of vulnerabilities to losses of multiple kinds arising from any identifiable threat to some dimension of well-being. For example, it is difficult to imagine persons being vulnerable to loss of property and possessions without being vulnerable to all the economic and psychological consequences of homelessness and displacement. The ethically appropriate discharge of public health planning responsibilities, therefore, encompasses a duty to anticipate both the range of distinct types of loss that the subpopulations might experience and the overlapping causal mechanisms by which losses occasioned by a disaster are made greater and more difficult to mitigate because of the preexisting vulnerabilities of those subpopulations. The minimal expression of such a duty involves a responsibility to identify those particular populations who are at increased vulnerability to losses above and beyond the general population and to incorporate loss mitigation and prevention strategies appropriately tailored to those differences in vulnerability into disaster preparedness and response plans.

Risk of Loss

During a natural disaster or pandemic, everyone is vulnerable to the various kinds of health and other losses discussed previously, but the challenge may be more substantial when considering subgroups. Certain socially situated groups, for a number of reasons, have a different risk profile than most other members of the community.

First, certain groups might face a greater probability of experiencing a harm or loss of a specific kind. They might have a medical condition making their adverse health outcomes worse or a limitation of mobility that reduces their ability to takes steps to mitigate the impact of a disaster.

Second, some groups may be more likely to experience a greater magnitude of a particular kind of loss. For example, they may be geographically nearer to the greatest impact of a natural disaster, such as a flood, or an industrial event, such as an accident or terrorist attack.

Third, groups with multiple vulnerabilities face a greater aggregate magnitude of loss in well-being because the combined effect of losses of various kinds is the likely consequence of a cascade of causally related losses. Those who are poor, lack access to transportation, are in poor health, and have inadequate housing are more vulnerable to multiple losses that can magnify the adverse impact on any one aspect of their overall well-being. The cumulative effect of such cascading losses can be far more devastating than any single loss to persons who do not face multiple vulnerabilities. For example, an industrial accident or natural disaster that destroys a home is bad enough for healthy persons, but for those who are already medically vulnerable, the loss of adequate shelter can expose them to new health threats that add to existing comorbidities. If persons who are medically vulnerable are located in rural or sparsely populated areas, geographic inaccessibility to timely medical care can make such an assault on health far greater than it would otherwise have been if all the other contributing factors to poor health outcomes not been present and if they had easier access to timely medical care.

In short, the potential impact of a disaster on some population groups may be far greater than on others, and public health planners should work to avoid unjust burdens on those who, by virtue of increased vulnerabilities, face greater than the population-average level of risk.

The experience of the poorest citizens of New Orleans during Hurricane Katrina provides a readily understandable example. The devastation of housing stock and the attendant dislocation affected everyone in the path of the storm because of the flooding produced by the break in the levees, but, for the poor, both the probability and magnitude of harm and the cascade of other harms were greater (Atkins & Moy, 2005). The poor in New Orleans, like the poor elsewhere, tend to live on property that is closest to sources of hazard. In New Orleans, their increased probability of loss from the levee break was a consequence of living on low-elevation land, where the probability of flooding would be highest and the magnitude of destruction the greatest.

The special vulnerability of the poor to greater risk of harm is not limited to natural disasters. The poor tend to live closer to other sources of hazard, such as chemical factories, power plants, train tracks and freight storage depots, gas and fuel processor plants, and landfill disposal sites (White, 1998). If things go badly, whether as a consequence of natural disasters such as a hurricane, large-scale accidents, or terrorist attacks at industrial sites, the very fact of their close proximity exposes the poor to a greater probability of a greater degree of harm than their more distant neighbors can expect.

Although loss of housing stock and dislocation adversely affect anyone in the path of a storm such as Katrina, being poor usually means being without adequate insurance to rebuild or replace damaged housing, and being poor means lacking ready financial resources or credit to maintain the necessities of life until assistance from government or relief agencies becomes available. As a result, the ability to recoup from disaster is far less for the poor than for more prosperous homeowners. Loss of housing stock, especially the loss of building structures within a whole community, usually means a greater likelihood that the source of employment will disappear as well. If there are no savings or insurance to aid displaced families in rebuilding their lives, the loss of a job is doubly devastating. Therefore, whereas losses faced by vulnerable populations might be the same kind as those faced by others, the impact on those who are more vulnerable by virtue of their economic disadvantage is both far greater and readily predictable.

Socially Situated Vulnerability Versus Natural Vulnerability

Socioeconomic disadvantage in all its familiar manifestations is a form of socially situated disadvantage. Vulnerability of the sort described in the example of Hurricane Katrina, for example, is not a consequence of some innate or unalterable natural characteristic of the persons disproportionately adversely affected by disaster. Such vulnerabilities are largely a function of the contingent situation of certain groups under alterable social and economic arrangements.

In contrast, increased vulnerability to a pathogen may be mediated by genetic differences that predispose some persons to earlier onset of disease, a more robust form of infection, poorer prognosis, more anticipated medical complications or comorbidities, or less capacity to respond positively to available therapeutic options. Such vulnerabilities may be thought of as natural vulnerabilities; that is, the increased risk, either in probability or magnitude of harm, may be a function primarily of some natural biological fact about the affected persons.

The purpose of this contrast is not to draw sharp distinctions between natural and socially produced vulnerabilities but rather to emphasize that increased vulnerabilities may often be a joint function of natural factors and contingent social arrangements such as economic disadvantage. Because the two interact, such possibilities for interaction should be recognized in the planning process. For example, decreased responsiveness to available therapies is itself a function of both biology and of societal investment patterns in pharmacological agents of one kind rather than another. This is also true of matters of prognosis (e.g., when genetic predisposition accounts for the first component of increased vulnerability but lack of access to timely and appropriate medical care or public policies that reduce the opportunity of some groups to avoid exposure continue the cycle).

Elevated Baseline Vulnerability

Regardless of whether vulnerabilities are primarily of natural or biological origin, or whether they arise from some combination of socially situational disadvantage and predisposing biological factors, they translate into an elevated baseline vulnerability. In principle, at least, some groups who are vulnerable to various types of losses occasioned by disasters can be identified in advance because of known factors that contribute to elevated baseline risk. This is not to deny the need for careful reflection and exercise of the imagination for identifying groups with elevated baseline vulnerabilities; however, some sources of vulnerability are readily predictable and thus more readily amenable to being accounted for in the planning process. Predictable elevated baseline vulnerabilities include economic status, geographic proximity to known hazards, previously identified genetic predisposition, ongoing environmental hazard exposure, and physical or mental disabilities (Shrader-Frechett, 2002).

In contrast, some persons are more vulnerable to hazards that might not of themselves be readily predictable as sources of increased risk based on known preexisting group characteristics. Victims of terrorist acts, for example, are not always an easily identifiable group. However much planning and thought might be given to possible terrorist attack sites, the many imaginable sites that a terrorist might choose still present a large impediment to accurate prediction. Likewise, neither the particular instrument of terror nor its hazards lend themselves to complete and comprehensive planning to protect those exposed. Nonetheless, it is known that firefighters and police, recovery workers, health care providers, and volunteer responders will face special risks in the event of a terrorist attack. These will likely be in the form of environmental hazards ranging from pathogens to radiation to respiratory particulate matter. Even then, health officials may not have an adequate epidemiologic basis for knowing the long-term vulnerabilities of those exposed.

The implication for persons involved in both the planning and response stage is that they have a duty to anticipate those who, by virtue of some group characteristics, are at increased vulnerability for losses of various kinds, as well as a duty after the fact to monitor and attend to the range of potential long-term vulnerabilities for which any reasonable effort at anticipation may still fail to identify in advance.

Cascading Losses and Fine-Grained Variations in Vulnerability

It bears repeating that vulnerability to a loss of one kind rarely, if ever, travels alone. The additional vulnerability of certain groups may be a function of the fact that vulnerabilities that arise with respect to one aspect of their members' individual well-being not only magnify the probability and magnitude of potential harm (e.g., to physical health), but can also create additional vulnerabilities in the process. Increased levels of vulnerability to health or economic harm, like social disadvantages generally, interact, compound, and perpetuate one another. Being poor is a risk factor for environmentally mediated and medically unattended ill health, lack of cognitive development at crucial stages of human maturation, and increased vulnerability to violence and lack of physical security (Ben-Shlomo & Kuth, 2002). Being sick or having cognitive disabilities is a risk factor for being poor, being forgotten in the public health planning process, being more difficult to incorporate adequately in any rescue or disaster response plan, and living in substandard or dangerous housing conditions (Kawachi, Kennedy, & Wilkinson, 1999). Moreover, being sick, being poor, or having cognitive disabilities does not establish a one-size-fits-all standard of vulnerability for anyone who falls within the relevant group label. Being poor where agricultural abundance is the norm makes one less vulnerable to loss than being poor where everyone lives close to the edge of starvation.

Being poor is less of a risk factor for sustaining unrecoverable losses when a system of medical care is accessible and is independent of individual ability to pay. Being poor matters most when many of the goods necessary for life and for survival of a disaster are made available only on the basis of the ability to pay. Being sick similarly admits of variations in the degree of vulnerability to other harms, including loss of economic security and limitations on mobility.

Availability of public assistance programs or accessible public transportation not only changes the standard of living for the sick in the course of their ordinary lives but also provides some additional hedge or buffer against a cascade of losses when disasters affect the population at large.

Those things that can be changed in the equation of how much unjust, disproportionate risk and burden of harm will fall on certain predictable subpopulations are the background social, economic, and infrastructural conditions that, if configured differently, would have reduced the vulnerability some face in a disaster affecting a community. Disadvantage takes many forms and arises out of lack of well-being or a secure means to the pursuit of well-being in its many dimensions.

When multiple dimensions of well-being are adversely affected through multiple causal pathways, and especially when those so affected have little hope of improving their situation, there arise the makings of systematic disadvantage. Those who are systematically disadvantaged not only live in conditions of diminished well-being but also remain permanently at risk of a worsening of their condition.

Those who command a proportionately greater share of the community's economic resources are better off, not simply in virtue of having a higher standard of living, but also in having disproportionate influence in public affairs, augmented bargaining power in private transactions, and the full measure of respect and esteem of others. Indeed, the worst off may have little option but to do the hardest work, with the greatest threat to health and safety, at the least convenient times, with the greatest risk of ruin by a turn of bad fortune, and for wages that can never raise them above their current state (Powers & Faden, 2006).

The challenge in planning so that unfair or unjust risks and burdens do not fall disproportionately heavily on some groups is to study and appreciate the complex causal pathways to harm and consider within-group variations. Economic disadvantage is one source of added vulnerability, perhaps numerically the largest source of vulnerability that poses challenges to public health authorities. However, many more such groups exist, including those portions of the population with various forms of physical and intellectual disabilities.

An Example: Persons with Cognitive Disabilities

Persons with intellectual disabilities or other medical conditions that interfere or limit ordinary cognitive functioning have vulnerabilities that expose them to a greater probability of harm and to harms of potential greater magnitude. Persons with certain forms of intellectual disability may lack the skills necessary to fully apprehend, process, and respond appropriately to warnings of impending hazards such as pandemics or natural disasters. The usual burdens faced by the general population in time of crisis are thus magnified among those who navigate the challenges of daily life more precariously, and often only well enough with the assistance of others. These differences present a need for planners to address specific ways that a disaster might affect the cognitively impaired (National Council on Disability, 2005).

The usual methods by which public health warnings are communicated may not reach this particular population; thus, they might remain in the path of a storm or flood when others have left before the level of risk had risen. During a pandemic, they might expose themselves to vectors of disease and pathogens when others have been made aware of the need to modify their daily routines in order to protect themselves.

In the case of more severe cognitive disabilities, a substantial percentage of affected persons may be in living arrangements where someone else is charged with making routine decisions about all aspects of their well-being. This arrangement brings its own public health challenges in an emergency when there is a need to mobilize and coordinate responses for large groups of persons with limited understanding and capacity to make voluntary decisions for themselves.

Persons with more moderate intellectual disabilities represent a quite different vulnerability profile for public health officials to take into account. Those with moderate cognitive disabilities may be in quasi-independent living arrangements, and whereas they might be able to function quite well within a regular daily routine, they may lack the skills necessary to cope with and adjust to novel and unfamiliar contexts. Some may not get timely information at all because their regimented routines make coping with daily life more tractable. Others may be more easily disoriented by situations that are manifestly difficult for anyone and, as a result, may feel unable to make quick decisions or take the necessary steps to comply with directives about matters such as evacuation or protection from a pathogen. Like persons without such cognitive limitations, they may feel the need to reconnect with others or forgo the pursuit of their own safety for the sake of family members and close associates.

In such cases, what distinguishes persons with moderate cognitive disabilities from those with a more normal level of functioning is often a greater degree of dependency and attachment as a defining feature of their lives. Dependency of this heightened sort can make the public health task of efficient response to mass health threats more difficult to manage. Indeed, the psychological dimension of any public health emergency can be as great as the threat to physical health, and the effects can be long-lasting and profound.

In addition, many of the challenges in dealing with persons with long-term cognitive disabilities apply to any population that is sick, dependent, unable to exercise a substantial measure of independent diligence for themselves, and situated in an institutional setting. One possible way to make the response tasks more tractable might be to geographically segregate some populations so that a more efficient operation can be mounted and one single, large-scale effort in identifying and responding to persons with cognitive disabilities would replace multiple efforts. However, any reasonable public health approach will recognize two striking failings in this way of proceeding.

First, physical health is not the only dimension of well-being that must be considered in public health policy planning. Social segregation, even if motivated by a desire for the health of those who lack the capacities to care adequately for all aspects of their own well-being, has proved to be a myopic focus on one dimension of well-being to the exclusion of others. The desire to live among others, to develop and sustain bonds of attachment with family members and others, to lead self-determining lives as far as their cognitive capacities will permit, and to participate in all the other social arrangements that add dignity and meaning to a life are wanted just as much by persons with intellectual disabilities as anyone else. The old, the sick, the frail, and those with reduced levels of cognitive functioning cannot be warehoused or shunted away simply because it solves a management problem if and when a disaster strikes.

Second, disaster planning and response are public health goals nested within a larger set of goals that necessarily take account of what is necessary to live a flourishing life under normal conditions of everyday life, and not just what is necessary for the best public health outcome in a disaster. Those things that serve public health goals well in normal times serve public health goals well in emergencies. Solid health care and public health infrastructure, forms of social insurance that prevent bad events from cascading into even worse outcomes, transportation design that facilitates mobility for all persons, and proper management of environmental hazards and their proximity to human habitation all serve the goals of wise public health policy in ordinary and extraordinary times.

Varieties of Vulnerability

Perhaps no complete taxonomy of vulnerabilities is possible; however, some useful distinctions can serve as markers for the kinds of things that public health planners and responders can take into account when thinking of their obligations to vulnerable subpopulations. These include distinctions among the elements of risk, among types of losses, among threats or sources of harm and vulnerability to harm to some aspect of well-being, together with their causally interactive structure. The International Federation of Red Cross and Red Crescent Societies defines vulnerable populations as "those at greatest risk from situations that threaten their survival or their capacity to live with a minimum of economic and social security and human dignity" (Jenson, 1997, p. 58). In many societies, women, children, minorities, refugees, the poor, and persons with disabilities are familiar examples of those having elevated baseline vulnerability to losses involving multiple aspects of their well-being, which, in turn, are likely to be realized through overlapping causal vectors.

Disadvantage, even systematic disadvantage, however, is no perfect proxy for vulnerability. There will be those for whom life seems to be going well enough, but who can, in a moment, become a new group marked by heightened vulnerability as a result of some unanticipated event.

The Moral Relevance of Vulnerability

Thus far, it has been claimed, first, that justice requires some special attention to those who are especially vulnerable to the losses occasioned by disasters and, second, that most theories of justice converge in that judgment. The following is an exploration of the question of possible justifications for such duties and how public health authorities should understand their aim with respect to persons identified as having a higher degree of vulnerability.

Prioritarian Justice: Priority to the Worst-Off

Some prominent contemporary theories of justice argue that the central requirement of justice is a societal duty to give priority to the worst off in any context that requires some distributive choice among persons when not all who stand to be benefited can be benefited, given resource constraints (Parfit, 1998). In some versions of this "prioritarian" conception of justice, the worst-off class of persons is defined by their distributive share of wealth and income (Rawls, 1971). So, by definition, it is the poor who receive priority.

Other theorists have generalized the prioritarian account of the job of justice to say that there are other ways in which the worst-off might be denominated, and, accordingly, whoever the worst off are according to some plausible alternative definition, it is to them that the most urgent obligations of justice are due. The needs of the worst off trump the similar needs of the best off simply because the worst off already have unfairly lower levels of well-being. Examples of extended prioritarian views abound. Children should get priority over the old because they by definition have had fewer opportunities for the goods that come with longevity. The sickest should get the scarce drug because their needs are most urgent or their suffering the greatest.

Just as prioritarian alternatives are limitless (Brock, 2002; Lockwood, 1988), so, too, are the practical and theoretical issues raised by adopting them as policy guides. One problem is the choice among prioritarian definitions. How do we adjudicate the issue of who is in fact the worst off so that that title earns them the claim for priority receipt of scarce resources. In the context of disaster planning and response, many different subpopulations have a plausible claim to be considered the worst off. However, few think, for example, that whatever prima facie arguments exist for protecting and rescuing children, they should lead to adopting a strict algorithm of doing so categorically at the expense of the old. At best, the prioritarian insight elucidates one important consideration in thinking about what justice requires. A counter argument against any temptation to apply the prioritarian principle mechanically is one that holds that citizens or residents of any political association have a right to some sort of equal concern and respect in the creation of state policies or a kind of claim for "moral equal protection" (Harris, 1988; Powers & Faden, 2002).

A further problem for the prioritarian argument is the fact that giving priority to the worst off—for example, the sickest, the poorest, the youngest, the disabled—is an essentially backward-looking principle of justice. It assumes that the job of justice is to remedy or smooth out the inequalities of the past, even if doing so means that the public health aspiration of benefiting more people is thereby undermined. For example, if we only treat the sickest; rescue those who are hardest to reach; protect those whose personal characteristics make them the hardest, most time-consuming to protect, we risk not being able to treat more who will live if given a scarce drug in a pandemic or rescue those who are healthy enough to save others and survive beyond the point of disaster (see the Red Cross definition of vulnerable populations). The prioritarian argument in its most extreme form might mean pouring an unlimited amount of scarce resources into policies and activities for which little or no long-term gains in health and longevity or other measures of well-being can be expected. Regardless of which priority to the worst-off might be considered morally relevant, it has limits and may be superseded either by resource efficiency considerations or a parallel commitment to something akin to the moral equal protection principle (described in the next section).

A final problem with the mechanical application of the prioritarian logic to decision-making in disaster planning and response is the fact that, however a decision is made as to who qualifies as members of the worst-off group, it is a rough and imperfect proxy for thinking about who are the most vulnerable. Vulnerability is relative to many factors, including threats to well-being born of the disaster event itself and more remotely linked personal factors such as economic class, disability, or minority status. Nevertheless, this context dependency should not ignore the often predictable association between increased vulnerability in a disaster and the preexisting patterns of disadvantage that make prospects for survival and well-being markedly poorer for some than others. To ignore this association would be to fail to learn any lessons from Hurricane Katrina.

Moral Equal Protection

The moral equal protection argument is based on the concern that strict priority to the worst off is suspect as a principle of fair public policy when the implications are a commitment to reducing the level of resources available to all for the sake of some. The problem is more than gross inefficiency. Even if following such a principle does not bankrupt or vastly outstrip available resources, it would be incompatible with some bedrock conception of moral equality, equal dignity, or right to equal concern and respect by the government of a society. On the other hand, the underlying intuition of the moral equal protection claim seems fundamentally right, but, like the core insight of the prioritarian family of justice theories, it does not seem to offer the final word on what justice demands with respect to those who are at baseline more vulnerable because of existing patterns of systematic disadvantage.

An added measure of attention to the special needs or risks of the various groups believed to be especially vulnerable in disasters might be argued for on grounds other than the prioritarians' desire to smooth out and compensate for past inequalities. Instead of thinking that the job of justice is the backward-looking task of pursuing strict equality of outcomes—such as health, wealth, or longevity—a prospective aspiration of justice might be to ensure that all persons can go forward from a disaster without spiraling downward irretrievably into a web of densely woven patterns of systematic disadvantage.

The dominant moral end of this nonprioritarian argument, then, is not compensation for the past, but reduction of those pervasive forces that shape the life prospects of some segments of society so adversely that the bad consequences that others can escape more readily can only be escaped by heroic effort and sheer good luck. This prospective surveillance of patterns of systematic disadvantage and heightened sensitivity to increased baseline vulnerabilities of certain subpopulations thus seems a better fit with the insights of the moral equal protection argument.

The end, thus conceived, is not special treatment or special benefit simply because they have fared worse than others in the past, but a governmental response that is calibrated to the demands of a genuine commitment to moral equality. That commitment is to the prospective removal of impediments that contribute to systematic disadvantage and heightened vulnerability not experienced by the rest of society. It would not single some out for added benefit in order to compensate for past inequalities; it would only ensure that none, as a consequence of a disaster event, is left in a position in which it is virtually guaranteed that an already bad situation is made both worse and almost inescapable.

Equality of Prospects or Status Quo?

The question remains regarding the role of public health with respect to vulnerable populations; that is, whether the aim of public health, even as it has been rephrased, is the elimination of systematic disadvantage, which would be a robust guarantee of comparable capacity to move forward beyond a disaster (or avoid one). Alternatively, is the aim better stated as something more modest; for example, to make all persons "whole" or restore everyone to the previous status quo, however much that pre-event condition might differ among persons or groups?

Endorsing the latter alternative implies that there is no obligation for public health or public planners in either the design or execution of disaster responses to have any impact in realizing the ends of a broader aspiration of social justice. Victims of disaster, for example, would be left with whatever access to health care they had prior to the disaster even if the added negative impact on health left them in a condition of far greater disadvantage.

The appeal of the status quo principle lies with the thought that there is something moral in an argument that puts the task of justice in this unusual context; that is, doing what public health officials would not be deputized to do in ordinary times. The logic of such a position, however, poses a fundamental question. It supposes that the end of public health is largely determined by its mission to do good and avoid some harms to the general population without any serious attention to the distributive aspects of its mission.

Although some public health theorists might accept such a conclusion as unfortunate but not unjust, a substantial portion of public health theorists and practitioners would not endorse the narrowness of that vision. By contrast, the vast body of literature on health disparities and justice-based arguments for public health efforts to reduce those disparities provides a near perfect fit with the claim made herein: that public health in ordinary times, as well as in times of disaster and catastrophe, is equally concerned with the distribution of health and other disparities in well-being as it is with a simple maximization of aggregate public health. These are large debates not resolvable here. However, the existence of alternative ways of framing the ends of public health in this kind of context illustrates the extent to which the way that priorities are set in disaster planning and response will depend on some fundamental moral commitments that are not yet resolved in public policy circles.

References

Atkins, D., & Moy, E. M. (2005). Left behind: The legacy of Hurricane Katrina. *British Medical Journal, 331*, 916–918.

Bellagio Group. (2007*a*). *Bellagio statement of principles*. Available at http://www.unicef.org/avianflu/files/Bellagio_Statement.pdf.

Bellagio Group. (2007*b*). *Checklist for pandemic influenza preparedness and response plans*. Available at http://www.bioethicsinstitute.org/wp-content/uploads/2012/12/Influenza-Checklist-English1.pdf.

Ben-Shlomo, Y., & Kuth, D. A. (2002). A life course approach to chronic disease epidemiology: Conceptual models, empirical challenges, and interdisciplinary perspectives. *International Journal of Epidemiology, 31*, 285–293.

Brock, D. (2002). Priority to the worst off in health-care resource prioritization. In R. Rhodes, M. Battin, & A. Silvers (Eds.), *Medicine and social justice* (pp. 362–372). New York: Oxford University Press.

Daniels, N. (1993). Rationing fairly: Programmatic considerations. *Bioethics*, 7, 224–233.

Gostin, L., & Powers, M. (2006). Justice and public health. *Health Affairs*, *25*, 1053–1060.

Harris, J. (1988). More and better justice. In M. Bell & S. Mendus (Eds.). *Philosophy and medical welfare* (pp. 75–96). Cambridge, UK: Cambridge University Press.

Jenson, E. (Ed.). (1997). *Disaster management ethics*. New York Department of Humanitarian Affairs of the General Secretariat of the United Nations for the Disaster Management Training Programme: 58. Available at http://reliefweb.int/sites/reliefweb.int/files/resources/2561747D821E0256C1256DB70053E6D4-undp-ethics-1997.pdf.

Kawachi, I., Kennedy, B., & Wilkinson R. (1999). *The society and population reader: Income inequality and health*. New York: New Press.

Lockwood, M. (1988). Quality of life and resource allocation. In J. Bell & S. Mendus (Eds.), *Philosophy and medical welfare* (pp. 33–55). Cambridge, UK: Cambridge University Press.

National Council on Disability. (2005). *Saving lives: Including people with disabilities in emergency planning*. Washington, DC: National Council on Disability. Available at http://www.ncd.gov/publications/2005/04152005.

Parfit, D. (1998). Equality and priority. In A. Mason (Ed.), *Ideals of Equality* (pp. 1–20). Hoboken, NJ: Wiley-Blackwell.

Pogge, T. (2002). *World poverty and human rights: Cosmopolitan responsibilities and reforms*. Oxford: Polity Press.

Powers, M., & Faden, R. (2002). Racial and ethnic disparities in health care: An ethical analysis of when and how they matter. In B. D. Smedley, A. Y. Stith, & A. R. Nelson (Eds.), *Unequal treatment: Confronting racial and ethnic disparities in health care* (pp. 63–75). Washington, DC: Committee on Understanding and Eliminating Racial and Ethnic Disparities in Health Care, Board on Health Sciences Policy, National Academy of Sciences, Institute of Medicine.

Powers, M., & Faden, R. (2006). *Social justice: The moral foundations of public health and health policy* (pp. 75–76). New York: Oxford University Press.

Rawls, J. (1971). *A theory of justice*. Cambridge, MA: Harvard University Press.

Shrader-Frechett, K. (2002). *Environmental justice*. New York: Oxford University Press.

Uscher-Pines, L., Duggan, P., Garoon, J., Karron, R., & Faden, R. (2007). Planning for an influenza pandemic: Social justice and the needs and interests of economically and socially disadvantaged groups. *Hastings Center Report*, *37*, 32–39.

White, H. L. (1998). Race, class and environmental hazards. In D. E. Camacho (Ed.), *Environmental injustices, political struggles* (pp. 61–81). Durham, NC: Duke University Press.

4

Public Engagement in Emergency Preparedness and Response

Ethical Perspectives in Public Health Practice

RUTH GAARE BERNHEIM

Introduction: Emergency in the Context of Public Health Practice

Public engagement plays a necessary and central role in addressing the ethical dimensions of emergency preparedness and response in public health practice, hereafter referred to simply as *emergency preparedness*. Public health officials, as government authorities and as health professionals, have the responsibility to actively seek and provide opportunities for public engagement in emergency preparedness policy-making and practices (Stern & Fineberg, 1966). Public engagement should take place in at least two ways: deliberation about the societal values and ethical tensions underlying emergency preparedness and consultation about the ethical aspects of specific emergency preparedness programs and activities. The primary role for public engagement in emergency preparedness is grounded in a number of ethical principles, such as fairness, utility, and respect for individual interests. These principles animate the practice of public health and are enumerated in the *Principles of the Ethical Practice of Public Health* (also referred to as the Public Health Code of Ethics, or the Code) (Public Health Leadership Society, 2002). Engaging all stakeholders in the community, including vulnerable populations at risk of bearing disproportionate burdens during an emergency, for example, is an expression of government's commitment to fairness that lays the foundation for the trust and collective action needed in emergency preparedness.

A distinction between deliberation and consultation grows out of two overlapping dimensions of emergency preparedness. Like public health practice in general, emergency preparedness has both political and social aspects, and although public engagement is essential for both, the goals, and therefore the approaches, to public engagement in each aspect may differ. First, as a fundamental and necessary feature of public health political governance in a liberal democratic society, public engagement in emergency preparedness is required in order that government authority and government actions have political legitimacy. Deliberation can be either an informal or formal process of communication among officials, experts, and community stakeholders to explore the differing values and interests of participants that arise in emergency preparedness. Second, for the social dimension of emergency preparedness, public engagement is essential for developing and maintaining the social connections and relationships between and among public health professionals and community stakeholders that are the basis of public trust. The social aspect of emergency preparedness requires ongoing consultation with stakeholders in the community about specific emergency preparedness interventions at each significant step in the assessment, planning, and implementation process. Consultation can elicit important information about the most effective ways to achieve program goals, as well as community support for emergency preparedness programs. Even if the primary goal of communication is merely the dissemination of information, growing evidence suggests the value of providing at least the opportunity for two-way exchange in any public health activity. Researchers propose that "(D)issemination is not an end in itself; its intended benefits depend on integration and implementation by the end users, who will also determine the relevance and usability of whatever is disseminated" (Green, Ottoson, Garcia, & Hiatt, 2009, p. 168). In addition consultation can strengthen and maintain relationships between public health officials and community stakeholders through the increased mutual knowledge and respect gained in ongoing, two-way exchange about emergency preparedness activities in a region. The appropriate amount, timing, and approach to deliberation and consultation depend on the context, practices, and values in a particular community.

Public health practice provides a general context for emergency preparedness activities, and public health officials' responsibility for initiating and maintaining public engagement is central to their role and to the essential services they provide. In their role as government authority, public health officials have the duty to protect the public from imminent health threats, as well as the broad responsibility to promote health through interventions aimed at the behavioral and social factors that affect preparedness and community risk. The 10 essential public health services, developed by a committee of representatives from major public and nongovernmental health organizations, illustrate the range of political and social responsibilities expected of public health agencies in ongoing, day-to-day practices in local and state health departments across the nation (Centers for Disease Control and Prevention, Core Public Health Functions Steering Committee, 1994). Those services that have particular relevance for emergency preparedness include political duties, such as developing policies and enforcing laws and regulations, as well as social responsibilities, such as "Inform, educate and empower people about health issues" and "Mobilize community partnerships and action to identify and solve health problems."

The 10 essential services of public health, taken as a whole, present at least two types of ethical challenges in the context of emergency preparedness that should be addressed through public engagement. One set of challenges involves the scope or breadth of activities that public health officials should undertake. For example, does government have a public health duty to prepare citizens for an emergency by addressing social factors—such as the unmet social and housing needs of the homeless population—that may put a community at elevated risk of harm in an emergency? Such questions of scope often are addressed in a legislative forum so that some public deliberation about emergency preparedness policies does take place through the political process (e.g., when legislatures pass new laws about altered standards of medical care during an emergency). However, there is a significant need for more public deliberation about emergency preparedness goals and values, beyond the current legislative debates, to educate, inform, and mobilize the community to consider, based on an examination of societal values, what other actions may be necessary for emergency preparedness. An example might be a community prioritization policy to allocate scarce medical resources in an emergency (Institute of Medicine, 2012). Deliberation in the public forum, which is a vital part of the understanding of democratic decision-making, is an implicit feature of public health's essential services related to policy-making and community mobilization. Public health officials should seek opportunities to frame community discussions related to emergency preparedness policies in ways that encourage reflection about underlying values, such as solidarity, fairness, and reciprocity.

A second set of ethical issues in emergency preparedness involves the means or choice of interventions deemed appropriate in any given situation. For example, in the emergency preparedness context, should public health officials use social marketing techniques to influence the social norms for individual behavior during an emergency, and should they draw on the latest communication science research about message framing and visual imagery to shape the public's values and/or risk perceptions in preparedness exercises? Questions of means such as these often are addressed by public health professionals in practice, taking into account the parameters set by political/legal institutions, community norms, and evidence-based best practices. Public consultation is needed to ensure that the goals of emergency preparedness programs and particular interventions take into account professional and community values and are informed by diverse perspectives about their likely effectiveness in a particular context. For interventions that involve social marketing, for example, consultation with community members and transparency about communication goals, message design, and outcome measures for evaluation may be particularly important to maintain community trust among community stakeholders and with public health officials.

This chapter explores a deliberative, evidence-based process for emergency preparedness decision-making that incorporates appropriate public engagement in each of the essential public health services, from diagnosing and investigating potential health hazards to evaluating effectiveness and researching innovative solutions to problems. A similar, iterative model has been described for informing decisions about risk characterization and management in public policy in general. This chapter focuses specifically on the ethical dimensions of public engagement in emergency preparedness, drawing on conceptual and empirical perspectives on public engagement as they relate to public health practice.

Public Engagement and Emergency Preparedness

The different political and social dimensions of emergency preparedness in public health practice provide distinct ethical perspectives on the role of public engagement. As a political undertaking, emergency preparedness requires at a minimum that public health officials, as government authority, prepare to use and enforce laws in an ethical way to protect the public in an emergency. This also includes preparing citizens to accept government authority and actions that may significantly limit their individual interests (such as liberty) for the sake of the public good. In the political realm, then, a key ethical issue is the legitimacy of authority and of the liberty-limiting and rationing schemes developed and implemented by government officials for a public health emergency. In this context, legitimacy might be understood as being in accordance with the political/social contract that authorizes the existence of government authority and the use of that authority for these reasons and in this manner.

Much is at stake for individuals and groups in emergency preparedness plans, such as who will receive priority for scarce resources and whether, when, and for whom travel restrictions will be put in place. Given the context of a pluralistic democracy, a fundamental question arises: What type of public engagement is necessary for political legitimacy, not only for the development of a course of action supported by the majority, but also one that is ethically justifiable and acceptable to citizens who, as political agents, will then have moral responsibility to fulfill their civic obligations during an emergency? In a democratic political order, accountability and transparency in governance require that reasons, justifications, and explanations for official practices be provided to ensure that the public can support such actions.

As a social endeavor, on the other hand, emergency preparedness focuses less on the use of authority and more on engendering social collaboration and public trust. It requires that public health officials undertake many types of interventions, such as mobilizing social networks to distribute emergency planning information to families with special needs or providing translators for culturally appropriate consultation with immigrants who do not speak English. The goal of public engagement in this sphere is to build the civic infrastructure and social capital that communities need to anticipate, assess, and manage threats during uncertain and changing conditions. Ethical questions arising out of the professional–community relationships are at issue in this realm and include the following:

- What types of partnerships and collaborations build civic, institutional, and professional trust?
- How much information must be communicated to satisfy the requirements of truthfulness and maintain trust in the professional relationship, if there is reason to believe that provision of some information may put some lives at risk?
- When should public health officials provide not just factual information but also persuasive messages to encourage people to act in certain ways, even when it may not appear to be in their individual interest to do so?

From a social perspective, engaging the public about ethical issues in emergency preparedness in a creative problem-solving process helps forge support of public health programs, facilitates social learning about how to make ethical decisions and act collectively, and leads to collaborative relationships and social cohesion among and with community stakeholders. For this, approaches to ethical engagement might include communication around narratives about citizen leaders acting altruistically, empathetic messages of concern for those at particular risk in an emergency, accounts of health emergencies in the community's history and the way citizens acted collectively in those emergencies, and risk communication messages. Engagement might take the form of messages and education in the mass media or newer approaches that provide ways to respond, such as the use of social media (Merchant, Elmer, & Laurie, 2011), social networking websites, blogs, micro-blogs such as Twitter, and creative media such as Photovoice (Catalani & Minkler, 2010).

Although a broad range of methods for public engagement are described in the literature, distinctions among the various mechanisms are not well-defined in theory or practice. Rowe and Frewer (2005) list more than 30 public engagement techniques, from citizen panels and juries to community forums, town hall meetings, and computer-based techniques, each of which have varying levels of structure and formality. On the basis of the way information flows between sponsors and participants, I differentiate these techniques into three groups: communication, consultation, and community participation. In communication, information flows one way from sponsors to the public; in consultation, information (usually considered citizen opinions) flows from the public to the sponsors with no formal dialog; and, in participation, information is exchanged between sponsors and public. Other factors to differentiate the various engagement techniques include intention or objective of the engagement (e.g., education, input, consensus), participants (citizens, community representatives, leaders, experts), structure (formal or informal), and outcome (e.g., whether there is a specific decision or choice to be made). These distinctions may be helpful in planning emergency preparedness strategies. The type of engagement mechanism that is appropriate in emergency preparedness will depend on the goal of engagement (i.e., is engagement a political or social undertaking?) and the particular community context (Delli Carpini, Cook, & Jacobs, 2004; Papadopoulos & Warin, 2007; Roberts, 2004).

The following case scenario, which was developed with local and state public health officials at numerous national meetings during the past 5 years, illustrates some questions likely to arise in emergency preparedness for which public engagement is needed.

Case Study

During the first week of classes in September at a major university (20,000 students), a graduate student who recently arrived in the United States was admitted to the university hospital with severe respiratory illness. Before entering the United States on an air carrier into Dulles International Airport, the student had visited his elderly father in a hospital in Vietnam. Several days after entering the United States, the student developed upper respiratory symptoms, rapidly progressing to pneumonia and respiratory failure. After one week of hospitalization, the student was still in critical condition, not responding to any treatment. Meanwhile, three other students who live in the same international dormitory with the student developed respiratory symptoms. Most of the younger ill students appear to be relatively stable, although not responding to antibiotics. Diagnostic test results for all patients were nonspecific but were negative for influenza.

At the end of one more week, the respiratory illness appears to be spreading more rapidly. The hospital emergency room (ER) and Student Health Center have several staff members calling in sick, apparently with influenza-like symptoms. Student Health and the hospital ER also report increases in the number of patients with respiratory symptoms. They have sent many of them home with the usual recommendations for fluids or antipyretics. In addition, the hospital has admitted 10 more students and university staff members with severe respiratory illness. Of these, five have been admitted to the intensive care unit, and one death has occurred (a 2-year-old child whose parent works at the university).

The university hospital epidemiologist and nursing staff, working with Student Health, have collected information on all patients and hospital staff who have had respiratory symptoms. Laboratory results are negative for influenza.

University health staff members have reported the cases to the local health department, and the health department has conducted an epidemiologic analysis that suggests person-to-person spread of infection. As local health officer, you have reviewed the results of clinical and epidemiologic analysis and are concerned about the risk to your community.

Should you call for a voluntary quarantine for the university, or, alternately, should you impose quarantine of students who live in the affected dormitories? Should you notify the public, and, if so, what should you say?

The following questions, in both the political and social realm, are embedded in this short scenario:

- Can the use of governmental authority to impose quarantine be publicly justified (political)?
- What information should be presented to the community in this situation, if any (political and social)?
- What types of public engagement should have taken place in the community before this situation occurred so that public health officials and the community could come to an understanding about the deeper political values and tensions at stake in imposing quarantine in this situation (political)?
- What social marketing programs or risk communication strategies could have been developed in consultation with the public before the outbreak to prepare the public for an infectious disease outbreak (political and social)?

Public health officials can draw on public health ethics to engage the public in questions like these. Public health ethics, as a normative enterprise, can provide frameworks and principles to explore the public's understanding of the fundamental societal values that underlie the questions and that characterize the relationships and interactions between public health professionals and individuals in emergency preparedness. For political undertakings in emergency preparedness, for example, public engagement should generally take place using a deliberative model. This implies active participation of, and two-way information flow between, officials and the public, with explicit discussion about the ethical principles in public health that are in tension. Public engagement for emergency preparedness social undertakings might more appropriately be accomplished through consultation, for example, by inviting community input about emergency preparedness strategies or programs at various stages during their development. For this process, organizational ethics frameworks, such as the Principles for the Ethical Practice of Public Health (Table 4.1) can provide guidance (Public Health Leadership Society, 2002).

Emergency Preparedness as a Political Undertaking: Public Justification in the Context of the Community

Emergency preparedness is embedded in public health practice and in the political process. Whereas public health is understood to be "what we, as a society, do collectively" (Institute of Medicine, 1988, p. 1), the locus of much actual decision-making in public health, including during an emergency, is in government health departments, which have broad authority and responsibility, grounded in government's police power, to protect the public's health and welfare. Law, with its foundation in society's political philosophy, provides the general framework for the execution of these powers and duties and also sets the boundaries on state power to limit individual rights and private interests. Within these broad parameters,

TABLE 4.1 Principles for the Ethical Practice of Public Health

1. Public health should address principally the fundamental causes of disease and requirements for health, aiming to prevent adverse health outcomes.
2. Public health should achieve community health in a way that respects the rights of individuals in the community.
3. Public health policies, programs, and priorities should be developed and evaluated through processes that ensure an opportunity for input from community members.
4. Public health should advocate and work for the empowerment of disenfranchised community members, aiming to ensure that the basic resources and conditions necessary for health are accessible to all.
5. Public health should seek the information needed to implement effective policies and programs that protect and promote health.
6. Public health institutions should provide communities with the information they have that is needed for decisions on policies or programs and should obtain the community's consent for their implementation.
7. Public health institutions should act in a timely manner on the information they have within the resources and the mandate given to them by the public.
8. Public health programs and policies should incorporate a variety of approaches that anticipate and respect diverse values, beliefs, and cultures in the community.
9. Public health programs and policies should be implemented in a manner that most enhances the physical and social environment.
10. Public health institutions should protect the confidentiality of information that can bring harm to an individual or community if made public. Exceptions must be justified on the basis of the high likelihood of significant harm to the individual or others.
11. Public health institutions should ensure the professional competence of their employees.
12. Public health institutions and their employees should engage in collaborations and affiliations in ways that build the public's trust and the institution's effectiveness.

however, there is much room for administrative discretion about how and when to use public health authority. Democratic, transparent decision-making procedures have been proposed as ways to ensure the appropriate balance between public good and individual rights in laws and regulations and in the use of government authority. Norman Daniels (2000) proposes an account of procedures called "accountability for reasonableness."

An ethics framework for public health developed previously by the author and colleagues (Childress & Bernheim 2003, 2008) provides the basis for the proposal that public engagement is a fundamental requirement of emergency preparedness activities, given the ethical tensions that arise among society's core values in emergency preparedness. The framework is a principle-based, process-oriented approach that sets out presumptions about appropriate government public health roles and interventions in a liberal, pluralistic, democratic society and identifies the conditions that must be met to rebut the presumptions. The presumptions emerge from an understanding of society's core values (i.e., "public philosophy" [Sandel, 1996]) as expressed through its constitution, laws, and policies, as well as through its cultural narratives, myths, and social practices. For example, if a society's public philosophy establishes a presumption in favor of individual liberty, as many believe the US tradition does, then liberty would be one of the core values presumed to have the greatest weight when balancing it with another value at stake. This presumption would then provide the starting point for deliberation about the appropriate use of quarantine in a public health emergency and about the justifications needed to override the individual's liberty interests and impose quarantine. Public engagement is required as part of the political process through which citizens and leaders deliberate about what the presumptions are and whether the conditions have been met to justify overriding the presumptive values.

In emergency preparedness, when public health authorities must choose an intervention when more than one is legally permissible and fundamental sociocultural values are in tension, they should do so based on values and presumptions as understood in the specific community at any given time. For instance, when deciding to detain a noncompliant infectious patient under the due process framework in state law and policy, public health officials should offer public justification for taking coercive, liberty-limiting actions for this patient in this context. Real-time decisions are socially situated in particular communities; thus, accountability requires articulating and explaining reasons to members of particular communities to ensure that the community can support such actions.

To justify an action that overrides important societal values, such as liberty, in order to achieve public health goals, the framework offers a set of justificative conditions, which include demonstrating that the action is likely to be effective and that it is necessary, proportional, impartial, and the least restrictive possible given the circumstances. In any real situation, whether a particular decision can be justified and deemed necessary or impartial will be based on professional judgment and interpretation of values in that particular context. During an emergency, public engagement might not be possible. Therefore, officials must be prepared to act on the basis of knowledge they gained beforehand about societal values and the decisions that would be acceptable to the particular community, so that later they are prepared to offer public reasons for their actions.

Accountability and transparency with the public are required because each participant in the political community has a stake in the public good and in society's core values that are sometimes overridden. Accountability is crucial before, during, and after the emergency for a number of reasons related to political legitimacy. Accountability respects the community's political autonomy as a "self-ruling" collective, out of which grow respect for individual human beings and their rights and well-being, fundamental concern for others who are in the same political institution (i.e., with common vulnerabilities and dependencies), and faithfulness to well-sculpted political roles and expectations. Accountability can replace or be thought of as a surrogate for a voter-centric understanding of consent as the conceptual core of political legitimacy—the idea that government is morally justified in exercising political authority and does so in a way that respects the public's understanding and expectations of political institutions developed over time.

One political theorist emphasizes the responsibility of public authorities to reflect the moral understanding of the group in whose name a decision is being made and to justify decisions in a way the public will find persuasive by pointing out that moral judgments, unlike scientific judgments, are "everyone's job" in society (Nagel, 1995). In emergency preparedness, then, public health officials must create opportunities for deliberation in order to explore the community's values and the rhetorical strategies that will be accepted during emergencies. In contrast to the public's response to HIV/AIDS, when in the early years of the epidemic a politically organized gay community played an important role in initiating public discussion (Bayer, 1995), for emergency preparedness there may not be any one stakeholder group in a community that will generate public discussion. Public officials, then, should initiate public engagement of some type so that they can prepare themselves to act in an emergency with an understanding of the moral perspectives of the particular community. As with a fire drill, government leaders and communities together must practice for an emergency that carries risk of great harm and implicates fundamental values, and this includes planning and practicing how to make and justify value-laden decisions.

In a pluralistic, liberal democracy, a two-way, deliberative method is appropriate to explore ethical tensions that occur in emergency preparedness, such as policies for the allocation of scarce resources. Deliberation in the political realm can be thought of as "debate and discussion aimed at producing reasonable, well-informed opinions in which participants are willing to revise preferences in light of discussion, new information, and claims made by fellow participants" (Chambers, 2003, p. 309). The potential benefits of a deliberative approach have been further described: "Although few adhere to the view that deliberation inevitably leads to consensus, many believe that deliberation under the right conditions will have a tendency to broaden perspectives, promote toleration and understanding between groups, and generally encourage a public-spirited attitude" (Chambers, 2003, p. 318).

Some believe that the proliferation of deliberative procedures in recent decades is related to evidence that public participation enhances political legitimacy. Understanding the process for achieving legitimacy has particular significance for preparing leaders to be effective in emergency preparedness. From a social psychology perspective, legitimacy can be understood as an "an internal value that is linked to personal feelings of obligation and responsibility to others" (Tyler, 2006, p. 390). From a political perspective, legitimacy is "a psychological property of an authority, institution, or social arrangement that leads those connected to it to believe that it is appropriate, proper, and just" (Tyler, 2006, p. 375). Research shows that people are not influenced simply by power and that "authorities and institutions are legitimated by the manner in which they make decisions and exercise authority" (Tyler, 2006, p. 394). Legitimacy, therefore, often is derived more from people's judgments about whether authorities use fair or ethical procedures and less from their judgments about the actual fairness or favorableness of the decisions. Legitimacy is particularly important during periods of scarcity and conflict. "Because of legitimacy, people feel that they ought to defer to decisions and rules, following them voluntarily out of obligation rather than out of fear of punishment or anticipation of reward. Being legitimate is important to the success of authorities, institutions, and institutional arrangements, since it is difficult to exert influence over others based solely upon the possession and use of power" (Tyler, 2006, p. 375).

For the purposes of emergency preparedness, then, deliberation is a way to express and engender the reciprocity needed to elicit collective action rather than to enforce compliance through the use of power. It may be approached as an educational and open-ended process in which community members, leaders, and public health officials have the opportunity to articulate and deliberate about emergency preparedness policies and decisions and the values that underlie them. It may be thought of as a conversation that precedes decision-making, an imaginative process that goes beyond mathematical formulas and technical information (Buttom & Mattson, 1999). Normative conditions for such deliberation include two primary considerations: fairness (of process and in representation) and respect (for participants and for the deliberative process). Goals of deliberation might be broadly framed, for example, to encourage a public-spirited perspective on emergency preparedness, to promote mutual respect among community members and public officials through inclusion and civility, and to enhance the quality of future decisions by increasing the knowledge of officials and community members of each other. Although there is a growing empirical literature describing various public participation and deliberation methods, evaluating and generalizing about the value and outcomes of particular methods are difficult because of the many ways any one technique is used and the mediating effects of the larger social context in which it takes place (Butterfoss, 2006; Guttman, 2007; Irvin & Stansbury, 2004).

For emergency preparedness, communities should consider creating opportunities for two different types or methods of public deliberation: forums or town hall meetings, which are generally thought to be open, larger, hearings providing broad inclusive settings where community members present their positions and can interact with others and citizens' panels or juries, which tend to be smaller groups of participants invited or selected to engage in more structured deliberation. Each method will be described briefly to illustrate their different characteristics; however, communities must decide how to adapt each method to their particular social context. Forums and juries may be set up in innumerable ways, and evidence about best practices is needed, especially regarding measures that address the normative conditions of fairness and respectfulness. To maximize the value of both methods, publicity should be generated in the media to encourage further deliberation about emergency preparedness policies throughout the community.

Although public forums, public hearings, and town hall meetings create opportunities for wide representation and open discussion, the weaknesses of these approaches include the variability of voluntary participation, time limitations that restrict extended exchange, and potential practical problems that are difficult to predict and control. The latter might include the deference often accorded to political leaders and technical experts and asymmetries of power and influence based on individual characteristics (e.g., educational background) of certain speakers. In addition, whereas invitations and publicity can be widely disseminated in the community before the events, no mechanism exists to ensure broad representation and informed participation.

In contrast, citizens' panels, consensus conferences, planning cells, or what will be referred to as "citizen juries" bring together a group of randomly selected people to discuss a chosen policy issue. In these methods, participants usually hear a wide range of views about the topic from experts. Moderators ensure that proceedings are fairly run and that participants are given a chance to cross-examine experts and each other and ask for more information if needed. These methods serve to inform and educate participants, stimulate exchange of ideas, and inform government officials of public beliefs.

Proponents believe these methods offer a constructive way to present and examine public values and opinions, which are often transformed through negotiation during public deliberation. In public forums, such as juries, "the reciprocal requirement to put forward reasons and to respond to challenges will tend to eliminate irrational preferences based on false empiric beliefs, morally repugnant preferences that no one is willing to advance in the public arena, and narrowly self-regarding preferences" (Smith & Wales, 2000, p. 53). One limitation of juries, however, is that although they aim for broad representation, problems arise in defining representation of the population in such a small group (usually 12–25 people). Nevertheless, several features make juries well-suited for engaging the public in the ethical values at stake in emergency preparedness: the inclusion of high levels of expertise, the neutrality and diverse representation of the jurors, and the process by which all participants voice positions and defend their views in a forum that sets conditions of respectfulness and civility.

By using both open public forums and smaller representational groups such as citizen juries, public health officials and communities can explore their presumptions about the societal values at stake in emergency preparedness, the way these values should inform decisions about particular emergency preparedness programs, and the justifications that can be offered by public health authorities for their emergency preparedness actions. Deliberative methods are only tools, however, and their effectiveness depends on factors related to procedural fairness, such as ensuring the involvement or representation of stakeholders and carefully managing the deliberative process through such mechanisms as setting agendas and establishing time limits to ensure a fair hearing of all participants.

Public Engagement as a Social Undertaking: Public Trust in the Context of Professional–Public Relationships

The process of actually preparing a community for an emergency is essentially a social undertaking that involves creating and strengthening relationships, partnerships, and collaborations throughout the community. Evidence from environmental policy-making over the past three decades, when government agencies have included the public in a wide range of environmental decisions, shows that public participation, when done well, can lead to "better results in terms of environmental quality and other social objectives . . ." and "also can enhance trust and understanding among parties." (Dietz & Stern, 2008, p. 2). On the basis of cases and evidence, an expert panel recently recommended: "Public participation should be fully incorporated into environmental assessment and decision-making processes, and it should be recognized by government agencies and other organizers of the processes as a requisite of effective action, not merely a formal procedural requirement" (Dietz & Stern, 2008, p. 2). Public health, like environmental decision-making, involves choices about values as well as analyses of scientific and technical data, and it similarly often requires actions by, and changes in, behaviors of community stakeholders, including collaboration with other actors with diverse interests and cultures.

Thus, public engagement and relationship building, it might be argued, provide a necessary foundation for public health practice. The recent Institute of Medicine (IOM) report (2003), *The Future of the Public Health in the 21st Century*, highlights the importance of relationships built on common goals: "All partners who can contribute to action as a public health system should be encouraged to assess their roles and responsibilities, consider changes, and devise ways to better collaborate with other partners. They can transform the way they 'do business' to better act to achieve a healthy population on their own and position themselves to be part of an effective partnership in assuring the health of the population." (Institute of Medicine, 2003, p. 32). One proposal in the report is for public health to build "a new generation of intersectoral partnerships that also draw on the perspectives and resources of diverse communities and actively engage them in health action" (Institute of Medicine, 2003, p. 4).

Although the relationship between government public health officials and others is one manifestation of the complex relationship between government and individuals, it is a specific type of relationship because health is a primary public good, and many aspects of human potential, such as employment, are contingent on it. In this type of relationship, public health officials act not only as government officers, but also as health professionals to the community. Public health is an evolving profession, and, as a social institution, it negotiates with society the terms of its relationship to satisfy the profession's need for autonomy and society's interest in public service and accountability. "Society's granting of power and privilege to the professions is premised on their willingness and ability to contribute to the social wellbeing and to conduct their affairs in a manner consistent with broader social values" (Frankel, 1989, p. 110). Trust is a necessary feature and outcome of a professional–client relationship and, in the context of public health, has been defined as "the belief that those with whom one interacts will take one's interests into account, even in situations in which one is not in a position to recognize, evaluate, or thwart a potentially negative course of action by those trusted" (Institute of Medicine, 1996, p. 37).

Professional ethics in public health, then, provides an important foundation for emergency preparedness, much like medical ethics and the widely known Hippocratic Oath do for the practice of medicine. Recognizing the need for ethical guidance to engender relationships of trust with community members from diverse groups, families, cultures, and religions, the Public Health Leadership Society developed the Public Health Code of Ethics (2002). The value of a code of ethics for public health practice is readily demonstrated by the challenge of emergency preparedness in practice. One potential benefit of the Public Health Code of Ethics is that it clarifies the professional roles and values of public health officials and provides an ethical framework and tool to which professionals can refer when making decisions and communicating with the public and other public officials. Additionally, it focuses attention on the organizational context of professional practice in public health. Professional ethics in public health includes the norms and practices within the public health agency, which, as an organization, has an internal management structure that affects public health professionals' relationships with community members with whom they interact in day-to-day practice.

Institute of Medicine reports in 1988 and 2003 called for the strengthening of US federal, state, and local government agencies, and the Public Health Code of Ethics includes five principles that address the obligations of public health agencies. An organizational ethics approach to emergency preparedness and response draws attention to the role and the tasks of seemingly unrelated public health personnel. For instance, if public health restaurant inspectors have demonstrated competence and impartiality in their daily decision-making over time, they have built the relationships of trust and mutual respect with community stakeholders that are essential for social cohesion and acceptance of difficult community decisions in an emergency. The challenge for public health agencies is to identify specific ways to integrate an ethics process based on the *Principles of the Ethical Practice of Public Health* (Public Health Leadership Society, 2002) into the organization's activities, such as through quality improvement processes and program evaluation. An understanding of the significance of social capital and of a community's relationships for emergency preparedness suggests that formalistic mechanisms, such as political checks and balances, are not sufficient to generate the complex relationships needed for effective governance and social trust in emergency preparedness.

The 12 principles in the Public Health Code of Ethics, as broad statements about the values implicit in actual public health practice, implicitly acknowledge the wide range of shifting and often conflicting beliefs, social norms, and loyalties in the US political tradition, as well as the need for the principles to be interpreted and specified in community practice. Thus, the Public Health Code of Ethics offers no hierarchical weighting of the different principles, deferring instead to professional judgment about the weights and specification of the principles in each community and the appropriate balancing of collective and individual interests. The Public Health Code of Ethics highlights the importance of community as both a concept and a specific geographic entity. For instance, although it explicitly values the liberal democratic commitment to respect individual rights in public health, it recognizes individual interests within the context of community (Principle 2).

The meaning of community and the concept of public consent in public health are explored in a report on public health ethics by the Nuffield Council on Bioethics in the United Kingdom (2007). In proposing a corrective to the traditional liberal framework's individualistic focus in public health policy-making, the report explicitly adds the value of community to its analysis. The term "community" is used to express the "value of belonging to a society in which each person's welfare, and that of the whole community, matters to everyone" (Nuffield Council on Bioethics, 2007, p. 23). The report claims that the need for individual consent for public health programs is limited when consent would obstruct important public health benefits. The limitation on the need for consent is justified by the value of community. The report states that "[p]ublic health often depends on universal programmes which need to be endorsed collectively if they are to be successfully implemented. Although the initial liberal framework supports the promotion of public goods and services, it presents these primarily as ways of promoting individual welfare. Hence, it does not adequately express the shared commitment to collective ends, which is a key ingredient in public support for programmes aimed at securing goods that are essentially collective" (Nuffield Council on Bioethics, 2007, p. 23).

Similarly, the focus of the *Principles of the Ethical Practice of Public Health* (Public Health Leadership Society, 2002) on "achieving community health" and "obtaining the community's consent" does not reflect the individualistic notions that underpin medical informed consent in a liberal framework. Given the values expressed throughout the Code, community consent would be obtained through a variety of approaches to public engagement: ensuring an opportunity for input from the community members (Principle 3), seeking the information needed from community stakeholders to implement effective policies and programs (Principle 5), advocating and working for the empowerment of disenfranchised community members that would involve ensuring their voices were heard in decision-making (Principle 4), and providing information to communities and engaging in collaborations and affiliations (Principle 12).

Principles 6 and 8 of the Public Health Code of Ethics are especially relevant for emergency preparedness and suggest that public health officials should take the initiative to engage especially those with diverse perspectives in the process of planning and decision-making. The language of the Code, stating that public health professionals "should act," "should advocate for," and "should engage" calls for public health to actively develop strong community relationships.

Creating such opportunities requires engaging community members in many situations that are not organized solely for emergency preparedness in order to reach a diverse group of people in different settings in their daily lives. These might include activities that public health agencies routinely do for other services, such as providing education at parent–teacher association meetings, religious services, and social events. Engaging the community to build the social infrastructure necessary for emergency preparedness would require more than holding open town meetings or special consultations with community leaders and experts about emergency preparedness. The Code suggests that, through grassroots community dialog, officials and community members share responsibility in developing policies for emergency preparedness and that together they can integrate a richer understanding of the ethical and cultural dimensions of emergency preparedness plans and of their respective civic roles and obligations.

An example of an issue that might be explored in community groups is the possible response different groups would deem appropriate and respectful if usual funeral services would have to be postponed during an emergency. This dialog would explore various religious and cultural beliefs regarding respectful treatment of deceased bodies. The specific opportunities and topics for information exchange, called for by the Public Health Code of Ethics, would depend on the particular populations, cultures, and practices in each community. The goal of these meetings would be both to seek information that could be used to develop plans and also to establish a respectful rapport among members of the community in addressing a collective emergency preparedness problem.

Another principle of particular relevance for emergency preparedness is Principle 12: "Public health institutions and their employees should engage in collaborations and affiliations in ways that build the public's trust and the institution's effectiveness." (Public Health Leadership Society, 2002, p. 4). This principle emphasizes the importance for public health to establish strong relationships with every sector in the community, such as businesses, faith-based and consumers' rights organizations, advocacy groups for vulnerable populations, and nonprofit agencies. The Code suggests that actively developing the civic infrastructure to cope with emergencies entails a creative social process with two-way communication and collective learning, including social learning by public health professionals themselves. Engaging the public in emergency planning "provides ready access to 'citizens' wisdom'—lessons distilled from the life experiences of many and diverse people—on how best to tackle serious, unforeseen events" (Schoch-Spana, Franco, Nuzzo, & Usenza, 2007, p. 17). Consistent leadership by public health officials over time, grounded in principles such as those articulated in the Public Health Code of Ethics, is essential to building community.

Partnerships and collaborations can raise ethical tensions, including real and perceived conflicts of interest and conflicts of obligations. Public health officials, for example, regulate some community stakeholders, such as restaurants, and this may constrain options for collaboration. In addition, public health officials often have competing obligations, as in an infectious disease outbreak when there is a duty to protect the public and a duty to protect the confidentiality of individuals. One study quoted the following firsthand description of the tensions these officials have experienced in balancing their conflicting roles: "what captures more of a sense of our primary purpose, being a partner with the community, a public servant, or an employee of the government? You're in the middle, you're a bridge, you're a forced ambassador, trying to make peace" (Bernheim, 2003, p. 109). The principles in the Public Health Code of Ethics provide an ethical compass to address the tensions that public health professionals must face in collaborations and affiliations, and, taken together, they suggest that one primary measure should be, "Do they build the public's trust?"

Some evidence indicates that community trust influences and is influenced by the formation, development, and effectiveness of collaborative partnerships. Although there are innumerable ways to structure and define partnerships, collaborations, and alliances in public health, they generally share certain features and might be defined as "an alliance among people and organizations from multiple sectors, such as schools and businesses, working together to achieve a common purpose." Research suggests that the effectiveness of collaborative partnerships may depend on the particular community context of the partnership. Some important contextual features include the history of previous collaboration in the community, whether the partnership forms in reaction to a felt community concern, and the amount of social capital, which refers to the degree of social engagement of citizens and their related trust for each other and for the institutions in their community (Rousos & Fawcett, 2000, p. 369).

The Code envisions that public health activities such as emergency preparedness take place within ongoing public health relationships in particular communities and that this real-world context shapes the meanings and interpretations of public health communication and collaborations between officials and community members. Relationships are multilayered and unique to each community. Community consent for much emergency planning and policy-making, as understood through the Public Health Code of Ethics, takes place as part of day-to-day practice through the many and varied forms of public engagement that include informal and structured communication and joint problem-solving by government officials and community stakeholders.

Public consultation for emergency preparedness, therefore, should take place within permanent organizational structures, such as ethics committees with community representation, and by means of explicit processes, such as ethics measures that include community input in program evaluation plans (Bernheim & Melnick, 2008). This will ensure that professional and organizational values, as well as community values, are integrated in emergency preparedness programs and will guide relationships with the community. Through these structures and processes, health departments will decide the level or type of public engagement appropriate for the development and implementation of particular emergency preparedness programs and policies based on a set of ethical principles. For some emergency preparedness activities (e.g., policies on school closings), the health department will work with specific community partners, in this case the local school administration and board, to ascertain the appropriate ways to involve the public. For other emergency preparedness activities in which cultural norms are at issue (e.g., policies that will have an impact on religious services or funeral arrangements), public consultation might include seeking input from specific groups such as religious congregations and leaders through focus groups, surveys, or a special task force. Public engagement in each community is both an art and a science, and more study is needed to establish best practices in the field.

Conclusion

Public engagement is a necessary feature of emergency preparedness in public health practice. Ethical principles, such as those enumerated in the Public Health Code of Ethics, can help public health officials to frame the goals, methods, outcome measures, and systematic evaluation of public engagement for emergency preparedness. For example, to engage a particular community in an educational intervention about behaviors that increase population risk during a flu outbreak, a goal for community engagement could be to "empower disenfranchised community members," drawing on Principle 4 of the Code. The methods and evaluation for this particular community engagement activity then would be based in part on that goal. More evaluation is needed about appropriate methods for and outcomes of community engagement in emergency preparedness, particularly because, during an emergency, it may not be possible to engage the community in real-time decision-making. The challenge for public health agencies is to integrate deliberative, evidence-based decision-making, grounded in ethical principles, into day-to-day organizational practices that are measurable; these include issues such as quality improvement or accreditation processes (Bernheim & Melnick, 2008).

The case scenario about a potential flu outbreak described earlier, for example, illustrates the two overlapping dimensions of public engagement in emergency preparedness: political and social. The questions raised in response to the case scenario about community notification involve public health communication programs, social marketing, and risk communication. Both draw heavily on research from the fields of social, cognitive, and economic psychology to shape all aspects of the way information is presented to the community. Both programs also take place within the context of relationships that can be harmed by ineffective communication or communication that is not perceived to be truthful or trustworthy. In emergency preparedness, social marketing and risk communication are examples of interventions that not only accomplish a task (i.e., the dissemination of government information), but also provide a foundation for the public health official's ongoing relationship with the community. Whereas incorporating insights from communication science is appropriate for public health professionals in order to improve their effectiveness in promoting collective activity (marketing) or preventing panic (risk communication), ethical questions may arise: when does a "marketing" message cross the line from persuasion, which is ethically permissible, to manipulation, which is not? When does a risk communication message omit information that the public may believe it has a basic right to know as citizens? Although public health officials have responsibility to use their professional judgment to respond to questions like these in an emergency, their judgment must be informed by widely understood public values and professional norms negotiated over time with those whom they serve.

To prepare themselves to use their authority in emergency preparedness, as well as to prepare the public to accept and trust that authority, public health officials should integrate a consideration of ethical principles into their routine day-to-day activities. To address the communication questions, for example, a health department might establish a community advisory board for ongoing consultation about the creation of public messages to ensure that communication strategies adhere to ethical principles of practice as interpreted and specified in that particular community. Although the Public Health Code of Ethics provides a list of ethical principles that have been adopted by national organizations, health departments might also formulate their own mission statements and core values or principles, as well as their own goals and evaluation measures for public engagement strategies that are based on them.

This deliberative, evidence-based approach to public engagement will strengthen the following three features of emergency preparedness that are essential for political legitimacy, trust, and social collaboration:

- *Fairness*, based on knowledge about the diverse values, beliefs, and cultures in a particular community and of the justifications that most community members would find acceptable for particular emergency preparedness actions (e.g., the rationale for instituting restrictive measures or allocating scarce resources in a particular context).
- *Respect for individual interests*, which includes the individual's interest in the collective good.
- *Political responsibility*, based on an enriched understanding of civic obligations and of the parameters and expectations set by legitimate political institutions and processes. For public health officials, this includes the responsibility to initiate and provide opportunities for ongoing deliberation and consultation that are appropriate for particular contexts and for the communities they serve.

Acknowledgments

The author thanks James Childress and Alan Melnick for their valuable feedback.

References

Bayer, R. (1995). AIDS, ethics, and activism: Institutional encounters in the epidemic's first decade. In R. E. Bulger, E. M. Bobby, & H. V. Fineberg (Eds.), *Society's choice: Social and ethical decision making in biomedicine*. Washington, DC: National Academy Press, 458–476.

Bernheim, R., & Melnick, A. (2008). Principled leadership in public health: Integrating ethics into practice and management. *Journal of Public Health Management and Practice*, *14*, 358–366.

Bernheim, R. G. (2003). Public health ethics: The voices of practitioners. *Journal of Law, Medicine & Ethics*, *31*, 104–109.

Butterfoss, F. D. (2006). Process evaluation for community participation. *Annual Review of Public Health*, *27*, 323–340.

Buttom, M., & Mattson, K. (1999). Deliberative democracy in practice: Challenges and prospects for civic deliberation. *Polity*, *31*, 609–637.

Catalani, C., & Minkler, M. (2010). Photovoice: A review of the literature in health and public health. *Health Education and Behavior*, *37*, 424–451.

Centers for Disease Control and Prevention, Core Public Health Functions Steering Committee. (1994). *The public health system and the 10 essential public health services*. Atlanta, GA: Centers for Disease Control and Prevention, National Public Health Performance Standards Program. Available at http://www.cdc.gov/od/ocphp/nphpsp/EssentialPHServices.htm.

Chambers, S. (2003). Deliberative democratic theory. *Annual Review of Political Science*, *6*, 307–326.

Childress, J. F., & Bernheim, R. G. (2003). Dunwoody Commentary—Beyond the liberal and communitarian impasse: A framework and vision for public health. *Florida Law Review*, *55*, 1191–1219.

Childress, J. F., & Bernheim, R. G. (2008). Public health ethics: Public justification and public trust. *Bundesgesundheitsblatt, Gesundheitsforschung, Gesundheitsschutz*, *51*, 1–6.

Daniels, N. (2000). Accountability for reasonableness. *British Medical Journal*, *321*, 1300–1301.

Delli Carpini, M. X., Cook, F. L., & Jacobs, L. R. (2004). Public deliberation, discursive participation, and citizen engagement: A review of the empirical literature. *Annual Review of Political Science*, *7*, 315–344.

Dietz, T., & Stern, P. C. (Eds.). (2008). *Public participation in environmental assessment and decision making*. Washington, DC: National Academy Press.

Frankel, M. S. (1989). Professional codes: Why, how, and with what impact? *Journal of Business Ethics*, *8*, 109–115.

Green, L. W., Ottoson, J. M., Garcia, C., & Hiatt, R. (2009). Diffusion theory and knowledge dissemination, utilization, and integration in public health. *Annual Review of Public Health, 30*, 151–174.

Guttman, N. (2007). Bringing the mountain to the public: Dilemmas and contradictions in the procedures of public deliberation initiatives that aim to get "ordinary citizens" to deliberate policy issues. *Communication Theory, 17*, 411–438.

Institute of Medicine. (2012). *Public engagement on facilitating access to antiviral medications and information in an influenza pandemic: Workshop series summary.* Washington, DC: National Academies Press.

Institute of Medicine, Committee for the Study of the Future of Public Health. (1988). *The future of public health.* Washington, DC: National Academy Press.

Institute of Medicine, Committee on Assuring the Health of the Public in the 21st Century. (2003). *The future of the public's health in the 21st century.* Washington DC: National Academy Press.

Institute of Medicine, Committee on Public Health. (1996). *Healthy communities: New partnerships for the future of public health.* Washington DC: National Academy Press.

Irvin, R., & Stansbury, J. (2004). Citizen participation in decision making: Is it worth the effort? *Public Administration Review, 64*, 55–65.

Merchant, R. M., Elmer, S., & Lurie, N. (2011). Integrating social media into emergency-preparedness efforts. *New England Journal of Medicine, 365*, 289–291.

Nagel, T. (1995). Moral epistemology. In R. E. Bulger, E. M. Bobby, & H. V. Fineberg (Eds.), *Society's choices: Social and ethical decision making in biomedicine*. Washington, DC: National Academy Press.

Nuffield Council on Bioethics. (2007). *Public health: Ethical issues.* London: Cambridge Publishers. Available at http://nuffieldbioethics.org/wp-content/uploads/2014/07/Public-health-ethical-issues.pdf.

Papadopoulos, Y., & Warin, P. (2007). Are innovative, participatory and deliberative procedures in policy making democratic and effective? *European Journal of Political Research, 46*, 445–472.

Public Health Leadership Society. (2002). *Principles of the ethical practice of public health, version 2.2*. Available at http://www.phls.org/home/section/3-26/.

Roberts, N. (2004). Public deliberation in an age of direct citizen participation. *American Review of Public Administration, 34,* 315–353.

Rousos, S. T., & Fawcett, S. B. (2000). A review of collaborative partnerships as a strategy for improving community health. *Annual Review of Public Health, 21,* 369–402.

Rowe, G., & Frewer, L. J. (2005). A typology of public engagement mechanisms. *Science, Technology, and Human Values, 30,* 251–290.

Sandel, M. J. (1996). *Democracy's discontent: America in search of a public philosophy.* Cambridge, MA: Harvard University Press.

Schoch-Spana, M., Franco, C., Nuzzo, J. B., & Usenza, C. (2007). Community engagement: Leadership tool for catastrophic health events. *Biosecurity and Bioterrorism: Biodefense Strategy, Practice, and Science, 5,* 8–25.

Smith, G., & Wales, C. (2000). Citizens' juries and deliberative democracy. *Political Studies, 48,* 51–65, citing Miller, D. (1992). Deliberative democracy and social choice. *Political Studies, 40,* Special Issue, 54.

Stern, P. C., & Fineberg, H. V. (Eds.). (1966). *Understanding risk: Informing decisions in a democratic society.* Washington, DC: National Academy Press.

Tyler, T. R. (2006). Psychological perspectives on legitimacy and legitimation. *Annual Review of Psychology, 57,* 375–400.

5

Professional, Civic, and Personal Obligations in Public Health Emergency Planning and Response

ANGUS DAWSON

Introduction

Imagine yourself in each of the following scenarios:

Scenario 1. You work for a department of public health in a large city and, with your colleagues, have direct responsibility for responding to an outbreak of an apparently novel infectious disease with high rates of mortality. You have had little time off in the past few weeks. A number of your colleagues have contracted the infection and are hospitalized in isolation. There is much to do at work, and you feel that you should stay in the office this evening to try to catch up. However, you play ice hockey with friends in an amateur league on Monday evenings. You enjoy these games, and this is a particularly crucial game for the team. You feel obligated to both work and your friends. What should you do?

Scenario 2. You are a doctor who used to work in public health. However, 5 years ago, you decided to move to family medicine and now have a thriving practice. Your city has experienced an outbreak of a novel infectious disease with high rates of mortality. There is a shortage of doctors with any expertise or knowledge of infectious disease control. You have been asked to help out at this time of crisis. On one hand, you feel that, given your expertise and the fact it is an emergency, you should respond positively to this request. On the other hand, you know that this will have an impact on your family practice, resulting in possible suffering to your own patients and a likely loss of income. What should you do?

Scenario 3. You work for a department of public health in a large city and, with your colleagues, have direct responsibility for responding to an outbreak of an apparently novel infectious disease with high rates of mortality. You have had little time off in the past few weeks. A number of your colleagues have contracted the infection and are hospitalized in isolation. There is much to do at work, and you feel that you should stay in the office this evening to try and catch up. However, you are the sole provider for your 3-year-old daughter. Recently, you have not spent as much time with her as you would like. Should you work again or spend time with your daughter? Should you even be doing this kind of work, given its pressures and the risk of infection to you (and indirectly your daughter)?

Such scenarios are, of course, simplistic. Much more information would be needed to actually decide what to do in each case. Some are easier to resolve than others. We may agree on what to do in some and disagree in others. However, they are included here to show how conflicts between different obligations, and sometimes different types of obligations, are central to such cases and to our lives more generally. In this chapter, I explore some of the complex web of obligations relevant to public health emergency planning and response.

This chapter has two main components. In the first section, the nature and scope of the obligations relevant to the actions of public health professionals (PHPs) in emergency situations will be discussed. The section also includes a taxonomy of obligations structured around the way that they come into existence and a discussion of some objections to this description of obligations. The second section will apply this analysis of obligations to the context of public health emergency preparedness and response, with a particular focus on the PHP's duty of care. It emphasizes the inadequacy of the dominant model regarding the duty of care for thinking about public health emergency preparedness and response and argues for framing future discussions in the context of real situations and taking a wider set of obligations into account than those at the core of debates in the current literature.

The Concept of Obligation

This section contains a series of clarifications relating to the meaning of "obligation" and the nature and scope of the relevant obligations. The terms "obligation" and "duty" are used interchangeably here, since, where relevant moral obligations exist, they provide a reason for an agent to act.[1] Different moral theories provide different accounts of obligations and their justification. Although these complications should not be dismissed, this chapter is concerned with a different level of analysis.[2] Also there will, in reality, be a great deal of agreement about the obligations that bind us even if they are derived in different ways from any favored moral theory.

The second clarification relates to the nature of the obligations of concern here. I suggest that the relevant duties be thought of as being prima facie obligations.[3] This means that they are not absolute duties—that is, obligations that must always be carried out—rather, each obligation can be outweighed by other obligations in a particular context (McNaughton & Rawlings, 2007; Ross, 1930).[4] It is important to see that, on this account, the acceptance that one is under an obligation does not necessarily result in that obligation being something that actually does motivate an action nor does it imply that one ought to actually carry out that particular obligation. Prima facie obligations remain in force as obligations even if they are not actually performed, and they can be distinguished from the "actual" obligation or "all-things-considered" obligation that in fact ought to be performed given the particularities of the situation (Ross, 1930). On this view, all relevant prima facie obligations remain binding even if, given the situation, they cannot all be carried out at a particular moment in time. In other words, what is in fact an all-things-considered obligation does not exhaust or cancel out other moral commitments, although it does legitimately override other prima facie obligations (on this occasion).

A person's existing obligations are of many types and can be combined or can conflict in many different ways. This is because of the nature of the web of the obligations but also because of the complexity of the situations people are presented with. The key skill we need to develop as moral agents is the ability to respond appropriately to the reason-giving features of the situations that confront us. Being able to make an appropriate practical judgment requires sensitivity to the relevant factors, as well as flexibility and creativity. However, it is possible to identify and pick out key morally relevant features of the various obligations for discussion. What one cannot do is determine in advance which particular moral obligation will be the all-things-considered obligation that ought to be carried out in response to a particular situation.

In situations in which there is more than one relevant moral obligation, it is tempting to seek some prior ranking or ordering of the obligations as a means of helping to make decisions about which one takes precedence. A number of ways of potentially distinguishing different types of obligations are outlined in the literature and could be used as a basis for an attempt to establish some such priority.[5] However, I believe that any ranking of types of duties built on these distinctions will fail because there are no good grounds for holding one type of obligation to be superior to another in this way. All are prima facie obligations, and all can override or be overridden.[6] A similar point can be made in reference to a less formal ordering of obligations in relation to the individual, family, professions, community, or society. There is no a priori reason why extra weight should be given to obligations relating to the first of these, with decreasing weight as we move to larger social units. There should certainly be no presumption in favor of the obligations related to the individual always taking precedence over those to a community or of obligations focused on producing societal goods automatically triumphing over more individual-related moral concerns. For example, creation and maintenance of a public good such as herd immunity might take priority over respect for autonomy in some circumstances (Dawson, 2007).

The third clarification is that our obligations should be viewed as being complex rather than simple. That is, there is a danger in concentrating on simplified accounts of our obligations, discussing cases involving the application of either single obligations or, at best, cases of two conflicting obligations. Occasionally, such simplification is necessary in order to explore theoretical issues. However, this should be seen as being the artificial device that it is, and, by contrast, we must ensure that the discussions reflect the true nature of our social world. From this perspective, a person's obligations can best be described as a complex interwoven web of obligations, each one of different scope, relevance, and force. For example, each person might have relationships relating to family, friendship, work, religious or political commitments, neighborhood, community, and nation, as well as important considerations in relation to such things as language, food, or sports affiliations. The complexity of these social relationships is mirrored, unsurprisingly, by the complexity of this web of obligations.

We certainly need an account of obligations that encompasses all the relevant relationships that link individual to individual, an individual to other family members, an individual professional to an individual patient or a potential patient, and an individual patient to a health care professional. Such individual-orientated relationships impose obligations and have been central to discussion in medical ethics for many years. However, other kinds of important relationships and consequent obligations also exist, and many of these have been little discussed in the literature. For example, obligations do arise at the community, population, or state level when an individual has a relationship with a community, either as a citizen or member of that community. These obligations are of particular importance in relation to public health emergency preparedness and response because the PHPs involved in decision- and policy-making in this area must take into account relevant obligations that are distinct from those central to clinical care.

A PHP has, for example, an obligation not merely to an individual patient but to a whole community. Such a community is not just a mass of patients that have sought help from their health care providers, but an interwoven social group made up of individuals with their own projects, lives, and complex social connections. For this reason, PHPs need to take care not to intervene in an inappropriate way, and they need to ensure that interventions carry the minimal possible amount of risk given the end pursued. Not only is the "target" for the obligations broader in the public health case, but the relevant obligations are also wider in scope, covering not only treatment, but also protection of the population through prevention or reduction of harm. PHPs have a type of delegated authority, acting on the public's behalf to maintain and ensure the background conditions for a decent quality of life for all. Such obligations are central to public health emergency preparedness and response.[7]

Just as PHPs owe obligations to the public, in certain circumstances, obligations will also be owed in turn to individual professionals, both by other individuals and also by the community, population, or state. For example, the patient/potential patient has obligations toward the professional (perhaps regarding such things as informing the professional about any known risk of infection), but obligations might be owed by the community, population, or state to a professional as well. An example of this kind might be when the professional continues to work despite an increase in risk to that individual's health.[8] The community obligations may justify planning for emergency situations through the provision of training, ensuring adequate staff levels to prevent burnout, and providing equipment of sufficient quantity and quality to not only do the job required, but also to protect those doing it.

In summary, persons are bound by a complex set of prima facie obligations of various types, and PHPs will be bound by specific obligations related to their unique role in society. The difficult job for any moral agent is to negotiate a way through the complex web of obligations while critically reflecting on which obligations are of key relevance at any moment and providing a justification for the eventual choice and action of the agent. In some situations, it is clear that particular relationships and related obligations come to the fore; in others, tension can arise between our different social roles and related obligations.[9] These complex and conflicting moral obligations have particular relevance for persons whose work is related to public health emergency preparedness and response.

Different Kinds of Obligation

This complex web of obligations is not just random or arbitrary. One can impose a reasonable and justified taxonomy on them based on the way that different obligations come into existence. For example, a distinction can be made between natural or "general" obligations owed to all persons just because of their personhood[10] and more specific or "special" obligations that arise between individuals and groups for other reasons (Jeske, 2008).[11] Special obligations can then be subdivided according to whether they arise through the consent of the bound party, through contract, or as a result of participating in a particular social role or broader social practice. These kinds of obligations are particularly relevant here.

There may be some disagreement about which general obligations an individual has toward others depending on the individual's prior moral theoretic commitments, but two important obligations are those of *beneficence* and *nonmaleficence*. Such obligations are general because they are not only owed to specific persons, but to all.[12] Other general obligations might include respecting autonomy and taking account of justice. Such obligations come into existence because of the possession by the relevant party (in this case, all persons) of the characteristics that qualify for the status of intrinsic value (e.g., rationality, sentience, a certain biological constitution). Whatever the true set of general obligations might be, the important thing is that they cannot be set aside by any individual. A person can choose not to perform such an obligation, but she cannot choose whether she is bound by them or whether they are owed to others.

Special moral obligations can come into existence in various ways. Some are created as a result of acceptance by the relevant party to be bound by that obligation. For example, if I promise to do something, I voluntarily bind myself to fulfill that duty. However, many argue that all (or virtually all) legitimate special obligations are voluntarily accepted in a way roughly analogous to this model.[13] According to this voluntarist view, an obligation is binding only if it is freely accepted by the relevantly bound party. Voluntarists argue that this model applies even in the context of relationships such as friendship or parenthood. On this view, I have no obligations to my child unless I freely consent to the acceptance of such obligations in some relevant sense (e.g., taking the child home from hospital after birth).[14] However, such voluntarism is not how we ought to think of friendship or parenthood. This approach seems to assume that the ideal life would be one free of the "burdens" of the obligations that arise within the context of everyday social relationships unless they are explicitly and voluntarily accepted. This seems mistaken (University of Toronto Joint Centre for Bioethics Pandemic Influenza Working Group, 2008). Although some special obligations do arise from consent, accepting this does not entail accepting that all do so. Nonconsensual obligations are also a component of the complex web, a point that can be illustrated by a discussion of some role obligations.

The term "role obligations" has been used to define the duties related to "an institutionally specified social function" (Hardimon, 1994, p. 334). These obligations derive from the relevant institutional role itself. For example, being a parent involves certain obligations that derive from the particular social relationship, independently of the biological relationship. Role obligations have been further categorized into contractual and noncontractual role obligations (Hardimon, 1994). Contractual roles are those that a person agrees to take on or sign up for (e.g., being a doctor or firefighter), whereas one is "born into" noncontractual roles (e.g., being part of a family and being a citizen). The contractual obligations are those that someone has explicitly accepted by taking on the relevant role. Some of these obligations may be stated in a job description or a professional code, but such "contracts" do not specify the full range of the relevant duties; rather, it is the relevant social role that is central.

Voluntarists might insist that only explicit terms stated and freely accepted in advance are binding, although some may be more lenient and accept some implied terms. However, this legalistic model seems inadequate in terms of capturing the true nature of obligations. A key example of a relevant obligation is a doctor's or nurse's duty to care for a patient in need. In the role-obligation view, such an obligation is just part of what it is to be a doctor or nurse. This is not something that is an optional aspect of medicine, something that a doctor or nurse could decide whether or not to accept; by signing up to be a doctor or nurse, the individual accepts and is bound by the relevant role obligations. Although certain obligations that are commonly attached to such roles may well be optional, others will be at the core and stand beyond individual negotiation. The particular obligation to have a duty to care for patients, for example, is so central to what it is to be a doctor that it will require no separate explicit agreement. Another way to make this point is to see that the role (and its obligations) exist prior to, and external to, any individual's choices about how to behave in the role. To fail to accept the set of core standard role obligations will be, in effect, to either exhibit ignorance of the meaning of the relevant concept (e.g., doctor) or demonstrate a commitment to relinquishing the role.

However, role obligations are not fixed and can change over time. They are open to scrutiny and critical review from both participants in the relevant roles and from those standing outside them. Because such role obligations are largely established through social conventions, the nature of the roles, the professions, and the obligations can all be revised or even overturned as society's conception of particular roles changes. However, accepting this does not mean that the role obligations are open to individual negotiation and acceptance. Individuals can suggest revisions, but they cannot unilaterally choose not to be bound by core role obligations. In cases where they choose to reject a core obligation, they are choosing to renounce the role, not merely the obligation.[15]

Another kind of special obligations are civic obligations, owed to particular individuals and members of a particular civic group (a village, town, city, province/state, or nation). These obligations are a good example of noncontractual role obligations. Any participant in the relevant social organization will have the attendant role obligations just because he or she is a member of that social group. Many of these civic obligations come into existence as a result of individuals being born into them; they are not something that a person signs up for.[16] Such community or civic obligations are not merely the result of an abstraction from individual obligations within the community but are likewise related to particular roles. They are special obligations and are therefore binding upon individual members of the group, although some civic obligations may be devolved to proxies through the electoral process or the appointment of public officials with particular responsibilities. Such parties legitimately act on behalf of the community. However, civic special obligations are not voluntary in the way that obligations relating to participation in civil society organizations would be. I can choose whether or not to join a bowling club (and be bound by any related obligations); but, although I can choose to some extent which town or country I live in, I cannot pick and choose among the set of obligations that attach to participation as a citizen of that civic group. In summary, I can, in a sense, reject the whole package by moving abroad, but as long as I choose to remain within the group, I am bound by the set of related civic obligations as a whole.

Two general observations about obligations should be noted. First, discussion of obligations tends to place emphasis on cases of conflict between different obligations, but it is important to see that they can also reinforce each other. For example, my general obligation to prevent harm to other people in a particular society may reinforce my special professional obligation to care for you as my patient and vice versa. It might also mean that I have a stronger general obligation toward another individual if I have appropriate specialist skills and the capacity to, for example, save his or her life. In this sense, obligations may then be "additive" or reinforcing. In other cases, they may be unidirectional (a parent's obligations toward a young child), or they may be mutual (obligations between friends). In yet another situation, acceptance of one obligation by one party may create subsequent obligations for others. For example, society may have obligations to a health care provider and his or her family if that person accepts additional risk while working during a public health emergency.

The second general observation is that as an individual's relationships change over time, so does the set of obligations binding that person's actions. Becoming a parent, becoming a professional, or developing a friendship changes one's roles and thus the set of obligations that go with those roles. The fact that someone takes on a new role does not, however, necessarily mean that the new related obligations now take precedence over previous obligations. According to the view of duties as prima facie obligations, being a moral agent requires a person to be aware of the fluid nature of obligations, notice any changes in the web that are of relevance, and then take them into account in moral judgments and subsequent actions. The all-things-considered obligation (what we ought to do) can never be stipulated in advance because the person does not know beforehand what ought to be considered relevant in any particular situation.

In summary, PHPs will have to make decisions within a complex web of prima facie obligations that in turn relate to the diverse set of social relationships that constitute their unique individual life. In the three scenarios presented in the introduction, each situation will require careful consideration as to which morally salient features are to be given priority in the actual judgment about what ought to be done. Being a PHP entails a set of role obligations, many of which are not voluntary but fixed by this particular social role. PHPs' obligations are not just related to individual patients or even limited to just health care concerns; part of their role obligations are due to delegated civic or government responsibilities to preserve and promote the population's health. Sometimes the PHP role obligations will take precedence, and, on other occasions, other obligations (such as those owed to family or friends) will take priority. Determining what ought to be done can be difficult and can result in regret that we cannot do all that we wish to do. However, accepting this fact is part of what it is to be a moral agent.

Objections to this Concept of Obligation

A number of potential objections to this approach to moral obligations might arise. The first of these is a general skepticism about the existence of objective moral obligations.[17] An *objective obligation* is one that exists independently of its adoption or acceptance by a particular individual. The opposite is a *subjective obligation*; that is, an obligation comes into existence only when it is adopted by the relevant individual him- or herself. The root of this objection is the thought that the approach I have outlined here is seeking to change the nature of the moral. The voluntarist, for example, might argue that it is for individuals, not others, to decide the nature of the obligations that bind them; the only obligations that bind are those that are voluntarily undertaken (except perhaps for a very minimal set of general obligations, such as an obligation not to cause harm to others). This view, in turn, might be linked to a vigorous role for individual autonomy in morality; that is, perhaps moral commitments require prior reflection and explicit endorsement to be binding. Although a robust response to this skepticism would require a full account of the nature of obligations (and a background moral theory), at the intuitive level, one can see what such obligations will be like. For example, a parent may choose not to fulfill the obligations to care for his or her own child. However, this might be seen as a case of failing to fulfill expected obligations rather than choosing not to accept some optional obligations. Such parent–child obligations in fact provide a good example of objective obligations. Indeed, they are taken so seriously that when there is evidence of a serious failure or a continuous failure to meet them, others, such as state representatives, will in turn be obligated to step in and fulfill what is required by the relevant obligation. Individuals have a choice about whether to carry out their obligations, but they do not have a choice about whether they are bound by any obligation itself (where it exists).

Second, it might be argued that the obligations that bind persons in their various social roles are just too demanding, morally speaking. In a very real sense, this is true. The kinds of obligations discussed here will certainly be demanding in this sense, but it can be argued that this is what ought to be expected when thinking about moral obligations. Such obligations may suggest a course of action that an individual might not like, or they may require the sacrifice of things that are considered important to his or her life. However, we must avoid falling into the trap of releasing ourselves (and others) from obligations because they require effort to perform. Everyone might reasonably expect moral claims to require certain actions from them, and they cannot just avoid them by claiming that they are too challenging to perform.

Third, it might be argued that the set of relevant obligations described here is too complicated to be applicable in the real world. The picture of obligations as a web reflecting a person's relationships means that the situation faced by each individual will be a complex one. Each person will have the difficult task of ensuring that they have taken into account all the relevant obligations and made a defensible judgment about which action ought to be performed. However, this on its own is not a reasonable objection. Even if the relevant relationships and consequent obligations are complex (as they will be), that in itself is no reason to object to being bound by them. The obligations should be as complex as they need to be. Epistemic frailty about which obligation ought to be followed in cases of conflict says nothing about the existence or nature of any obligation. This epistemic issue will probably mean that differences in actual behavior will be seen between individuals responding to imperfect information or personal concerns. However, these differences reflect the complexity of the relevant factors and the difficulty of practical judgment. They are not an argument for moving away from an objective account of obligations. I suggest that an account of obligations is needed that reflects the appropriate complexity of the real social world and the web of obligations within which we live. Occasionally, PHPs or others may choose to adopt heuristics to help in decision-making. There is nothing wrong with this as long as they continue to see such heuristics as aids to decision-making rather than as substitutes for judgment.

The complexity of these obligations also does not mean that PHPs should give up on any forward planning. A number of different issues can be explored in advance, even if a person cannot specify exactly which particular obligation will emerge as the basis for actual action in response to a particular set of facts. The kinds of things that can be considered include the relationships that are central in the area of public health emergency preparedness and response, many of the moral considerations associated with these issues, and the empirical data relating to recent epidemics and emergencies. These factors can be used as a basis for gaining insight into the potential practical problems that are likely to arise and as a means of thinking through how planners can deal with them in advance of any real public health emergency preparedness and response crisis.[18]

PHPs' Duty of Care in Emergencies

In this section, I apply the framework proposed previously to the specific issue of the public health care professional's duty of care in cases of public health emergency preparedness and response. As discussed, PHPs have certain role obligations that are not all created as a result of voluntary acceptance by the individual professional. Some exist as part of what it is to be a PHP, and these are not erased or suspended during a public health emergency. One core obligation, which will be discussed in detail in this section because it is central to any caring profession, is that of the duty of care owed to a patient. When thinking of its application in relation to the actions of PHPs, it must be broadened in many respects. On the other hand, this particular obligation (like all others) is prima facie in nature and so can be overridden by other considerations. Therefore, it is not always the most important obligation nor will it always win out in a dispute with other obligations. The correct all-things-considered obligation can only be decided in response to an actual situation. However, the nature and role of the duty of care during times of risk and emergencies have been extensively discussed in the literature and merits discussion here.

Perhaps the most influential discussion of the duty of care in situations of risk to the professional is that of Daniels (2006), in a paper entitled "Duty to Treat or Right to Refuse."[19] He conceptualizes the discussion in terms of a duty to treat (referred to here as a duty to care)[20] that involves explicit acceptance by the professional of a certain level of risk as a necessary prerequisite to being bound by the obligation to treat. Using the example of the estimated level of risk of HIV infection that might result from routine and specialist medical care, the paper asserts that if the risk to the doctor or nurse is felt by them to be too great, the duty to treat can be legitimately set to one side. In other words, the obligation to treat only comes into existence as a result of consent by the bound party. Daniels (2006, p. 158) argues that there "must be consent to the risks involved in a duty to treat . . . professional obligations are acquired obligations, and acquired obligations in general result only from actions or roles one undertakes consensually." He suggests that there are limits to the duty, but the scope of these limits is linked to the idea of what the individual professional finds to be an acceptable risk.[21]

It is apparent from my earlier discussion that I think this approach is mistaken in a number of respects. The duty to care, as a prima facie role obligation, continues to exist whether or not it is accepted by the individual professional. Although this duty has limits, they are not those presented by Daniels. Rather, the limits come from the duty not being an absolute duty but a prima facie obligation, which will always remain binding even if it is not always acted upon. This obligation does not fade in or out of existence relative to the degree of risk or whether or not it has been accepted as binding by a particular individual at a particular time.

Daniels perceives the issue as being, "does an obligation to care exist where there are significant risks to the doctor's health from treating the patient?" He argues that the existence of the obligation depends on whether the professional has agreed to accept the necessary level of risk required to carry out the obligation. However, my answer to that question is an unqualified "yes." The obligation exists, whatever the risks. This does not mean that this particular duty always takes precedence over all others, although it is likely that it will some of the time. This is the nature of prima facie obligations. The amount of risk is not relevant to establishing the existence of the duty, although it may be relevant to assessing whether one is bound to act from it in a particular case. Of course, doctors are free not to submit to certain risks or take on certain patients for a variety of reasons, but this does not mean that they are not bound by the obligation to care. In such cases, they are, rightly or wrongly, choosing to prioritize other considerations.

Thinking in this way can also help PHPs to realize that they should not see the fulfillment of the duty to care in times of risk to the individual as being supererogatory, that is, going beyond what is required. Rather, fulfilling the duty of care toward a patient is carrying out a role obligation, and, as such, it is part of what it is to be a health care practitioner (although it may, of course, be overridden by other obligations). According to the view outlined here, if a PHP goes beyond what is "required" by her obligations, she is not doing what is morally required. For example, if, on this occasion, it is determined that a doctor ought to care for his or her own family, and the doctor fails to do so and chooses to go beyond what is "required" in relation to the patients, then the doctor is not performing a supererogatory act but rather failing to perform the morally required all-things-considered obligation.[22]

As mentioned previously, many of the special professional obligations can be thought of as being role obligations: part of a specific set of obligations that exist prior to and independently of their acceptance by any particular individual when that individual agrees to take on the role. Acceptance of a particular role implies agreement to all relevant role obligations, not just the obligations that the individual person finds acceptable. Some of these role obligations may be explicit and contained in such things as a professional code; others are not, but are rather implied (by, e.g., the nature of the social role we are talking about). One of the constitutive obligations of the role of being a doctor or nurse is that of caring for patients in need.[23] Although such a duty of care is central to the role obligations of all health care workers, in the case of PHPs, the duty is directly related to the core aims of public health itself, such as preserving the conditions for flourishing of both individuals and communities through the protection and promotion of both health and social justice. Therefore, the PHP's obligation to care can be considered as being broader, in terms of both scope and content, than those commonly discussed within clinical medicine. The scope is broader because the recipients of such an obligation are not merely individual patients but whole communities or populations. The content of the obligation is broader in that the focus of the duty is not merely on treatment but also on activities directed at harm reduction and prevention. As I argued earlier, the obligation to care is best understood not as a contractual agreement between doctor and patient, created as a result of mutual consent, but rather as a preexisting role obligation that is part of the core—even the very meaning—of what it is to be a health care professional.[24] In actual situations, a doctor might fail to fulfill the obligation of care either by deciding to ignore it or by coming to the reasoned conclusion that the obligation of care is overridden by an alternative duty that takes precedence in that particular case.

The prima facie duties of a PHP are multiple and sometimes conflicting. As a result, they often cannot all be fulfilled or acted upon in a particular situation. This is why what counts as a morally justified action is not determined by simply following a prima facie obligation alone. The required action is arrived at as a result of moral deliberation and judgment. Such moral reasoning determines what one ought to do, and, when successful, it captures one's all-things-considered obligation in that particular case. It is important to see that because the obligation to care is a prima facie obligation, although it may be overridden in one case, it remains a duty and may take precedence elsewhere. For example, a PHP might come to the judgment that an obligation to a family member takes precedence over the professional role obligation to provide care to those in need or to perform a professional function in the operation of an emergency response in those particular circumstances (such as scenario 3). In other cases, it may not.

How do we decide what we ought to do in such cases? There is no general rule or moral principle that determines the correct answer to this question in all cases. If the conflict of obligations can be resolved and both obligations fulfilled (perhaps by different persons or the same person at different times), then that outcome would be ethically best. For example, in the case of a conflict between an obligation to one's child and a professional obligation to care, the situation might be resolved if another caregiver (for the child) or a colleague at work can fill in your role on this occasion. However, such resolutions of conflicts are not always possible, and difficult moral choices often have to be made. PHPs should not make the mistake of thinking that simply because one obligation has been overridden in the course of following another that the overridden obligation has ceased to exist or was never a real obligation at all. If this were the case, then no moral conflict would have existed in the first place. The obligation that is overridden on this occasion will most likely take precedence once the force of circumstances changes. This aspect of our real moral experience makes the distinction between prima facie obligations and all-things-considered obligations useful.

Human nature being what it is, there will be times when a role obligation is left unfulfilled not because it is overridden by a more pressing obligation but because it is ignored. In other words, not all failures to fulfill obligations will be due to a decision to follow another (on this occasion, more ethically important) obligation. There are times when a conflict will arise between a prima facie obligation—such as the duty to care—and another competing consideration related to personal convenience, comfort, or preference. For example, you may prefer to play in your hockey game with your friends rather than carry on working, but such a preference will not cancel out a professional obligation to care in an emergency (see scenario 1). It is doubtful that such personal considerations will usually provide sufficient justification for choosing them rather than fulfilling the duty of care, but this does not mean that they should not be weighed in the deliberations about what we ought to do. In some cases, they may well be weighty enough to prevail.

Perhaps the most interesting and important situation of conflict between different considerations is where a PHP fails to fulfill his or her duty of care due to a reasonable fear of risk of harm within an emergency situation (e.g., risk from a serious, perhaps life-threatening, infectious disease). Self-preservation is itself an important and weighty consideration, one of both prudential and moral importance. Any potential conflict between one's professional duties and an increased risk of losing one's own life is a serious matter and difficult to resolve, as are the conflicts between one's professional and parental obligations, or conflicting obligations to different patients in a scenario involving triage. Again, there is no absolute rule or principle that will determine the ethically justified course of action. Each case will require careful consideration and judgment.

Having said this, two things need to be stated. First, the perception of a risk to one's life must be empirically well-founded; it should not be based on an unreasonable assessment of the evidence. Second, we might think that an individual professional does not have an obligation to undertake risk without adequate training, equipment, and support. If true, this in turn imposes an obligation on the relevant governmental or organizational body to ensure safe systems of work are in place. This is an essential background condition to the ethical assessment of the conduct of PHPs at all times and especially during public health emergencies. In a situation in which beliefs about risks are well-founded and supporting systems have failed to adequately mitigate those risks, individual PHPs ought not be bound to perform their professional duty. However, where adequate support is in place, the mere fact of an increased level of risk is not, in itself, enough to outweigh or cancel an obligation to care for those in need. The solution to this difficult issue is to ensure that appropriate and adequate preparations are made by all parties before the situation is faced, rather than running the risk of blaming individuals at the moment of threat.

Because it is known that many health professionals will fail to fulfill their all-things-considered obligations, this can be planned for in advance.[25] When the reasons people have for not acting from the obligation to care are known, they can be addressed as a means of maximizing fulfillment of the particular obligations society wants to see fulfilled. This may involve some substantial costs for society, but they may well be acceptable as a means of ensuring that health care workers are in position and willing to perform their roles when they are needed. This is part of the reciprocal nature of the relationship that exists between health care professionals and the population in general, and, as a result, the whole community is better off. Whereas professional ethics in public health emergency preparedness and response will often demand sacrifice, including exposure to higher levels of risk of harm, it ought not be a suicide pact. Nevertheless, if PHPs choose to protect themselves rather than assist others, there is a social cost to be paid. The community needs to be able to trust that health care professionals will be there when they are needed. This is why creating the conditions wherein professional ethics and practicality coincide is so important. PHPs should recognize and act in accordance with the relevant moral reasons, and this may mean putting themselves at increased risk in the service of others. However, more than their own moral understanding is necessary. They need to have a supportive and enabling environment, well-resourced and well-led, in order to be motivated to act appropriately.

Although there is good reason to believe that the majority of professional groups will respond appropriately (Morin, Higginson, & Goldrich, 2006; Straus et al., 2004), a concern may remain that, in a sustained and serious emergency, too few individuals will be willing to engage in required professional actions that might place them at increased risk of harm. Moral obligations can be enforced through the sanctions of a profession or the law (i.e., a professional may be removed from a professional register or may be prosecuted for failure to perform an action that is a legal duty).[26] However, moral and legal duties, for example, are not always coextensive. Enforcement of moral duties will have clear limits, since in many cases it will be inappropriate to compel behavior in this manner. For example, many will object to the enforcement of even a generally accepted obligation, such as a duty to care for a patient, when such action would increase the risk of harm to the professional. However, it is important to see that moral obligations do not require such sanctions to exist. The key sanctions in relation to moral injunctions are more likely to be such things as disapproval or blame, as well as self-evaluation and guilt. Such assessments serve as markers of culpability and wrongness. Often they will be linked to what is expected of someone when they perform a particular social role, or just generally what we would expect others to do for us in a situation where we would do the same for them (as friend, neighbor, or fellow citizen). Society provides certain incentives and rewards (e.g., greater pay or status) to ensure that professionals are available when they are needed. However, it is at least as important that society recognizes its reciprocal obligations toward these professionals and those that they care about. The performance, or even the prospect of a performance, of one obligation will create new and binding obligations on others. A society needs to fulfill its obligation to ensure that the necessary infrastructure is in place in relation to public health emergency preparedness and response in general, but also in relation to supporting PHPs in carrying out their role obligations.[27]

Responding to the Evidence and Planning for Problems

In this section, I discuss some empirical evidence related to actual problems that have arisen in relation to fulfilling obligations in cases of public health emergency preparedness and response. This is because when potential problems can be identified in advance, planners can discuss how they should respond to ensure that these problems are likely to be resolved. It is also important to contemplate what kinds of activities or actions should be encouraged and attempt to identify ways to do so. Discussing the available empirical evidence will help to ensure that the focus is not merely on ideal and abstract obligations, but that planners also consider the real difficulties that are likely to arise in seeking to attain the desired end of protecting the public in the face of an emergency. Two types of empirical evidence can be considered: (1) studies performed during or after real public health emergencies, such as the outbreak of severe acute respiratory syndrome (SARS) in Toronto and

Taiwan, and (2) research seeking to investigate how people claim that they would behave in contemplation of a future (hypothetical) emergency.

Three central issues arose in Taiwan during the SARS outbreak (Dwyer & Tsai, 2008). First was the concern of health care workers for protecting their own families from harm. This could have been better met by thinking of ways for hospitals to supply accommodation at work and means of communication with families that would not involve face-to-face contact. Second was the issue of child care. Again, it should be straightforward for hospitals and society in general to think about ways that conflicting loyalties to family can be addressed as a means to ensuring wholehearted commitment to professional obligations. Third, there were special concerns about the future fulfillment of important familial obligations, particularly in relation to children's future education. Again, this concern could be addressed easily, given sufficient commitment to thinking about the possible concerns of professionals at a time of emergency and ensuring that they are addressed in advance.

Another real issue that emerged during the SARS outbreak in Toronto was the tension and resentment caused by some staff "opting out," "not doing their duty," or "failing to take their turn" (Straus et al., 2004). Such tensions may persist beyond the point of the emergency, causing damage to teams that have worked together for many years. One issue that might be anticipated in such instances is how to deal with a concern of physicians (at least in primarily private health care systems) about the potential loss of professional earnings and the impact on their practice from the performance of their emergency-related obligations. Many physicians might be willing to perform their obligations but end up with significant financial loss as a result. Planners need to ensure in advance that adequate structures for reasonable compensation are in place so that this concern can be addressed.

In addition, future-orientated research examining self-reported willingness and ability to work during various kinds of catastrophes suggested that similar practical barriers exist, but most could be readily overcome (Qureshi et al., 2005). However, even taking such practicalities into account, the percentage of health care workers willing to work seemed to vary depending on the nature of the emergency in question. For example, the highest rates of willingness were for a car or airplane crash, snowstorm, or environmental disaster, and the lowest rates were for infectious diseases such as SARS or a radiation leak. This suggests that the perception of the level of risk will make a difference to the performance of professional obligations, even if potentially conflicting obligations, such as an obligation toward family, remain stable.

Given what is known about the way people have behaved in cases of public health emergencies and what is known about what they have said about the way that they will behave in such emergencies, it is important to plan for significant rates of absenteeism. What should be done in such circumstances? How bad would things have to get before such things as conscription of doctors and nurses are considered? We must reserve the right to do so, if the situation warrants it; however, this would no doubt be an option of last resort. Much can be done in advance, such as providing structures for adequate financial remuneration, transport to and from work, adequate child care, and accommodation at hospitals. Planning for such relatively simple and low-cost interventions is likely to significantly contribute to the willingness of health care workers to fulfill their role obligations. Such actions, taken now, will likely result in substantial benefit to the population in times of public health emergency preparedness and response.[28]

One final consideration is the reality of acting in the context of an emergency. What counts as an emergency is imprecise, but, given the account of obligations here, the facts relating to the particular case are important to the assessment about which obligations are relevant and which should take priority. For example, the amount of risk to the PHP involved in the response will vary, but so will the scale of the emergency itself. The response related to a one-time event (e.g., hurricane) will be very different from that for a prolonged event (e.g., infectious disease outbreak). Such factual matters will make a difference to the obligations that bind PHPs. For example, it might seem more appropriate to sacrifice a family commitment in the face of a one-time event rather than in the midst of a prolonged event. The other important factor is that preparation for public health emergencies must consider the fact that actions will have to occur in non-ideal situations with imperfect knowledge. PHPs must be prepared to act in a context of uncertainty. Training in ethics can be useful in such situations for developing a mature, flexible, and responsible workforce able to reason through what is appropriate and act with confidence to preserve and promote the public's health.

Conclusion

Persons involved in public health emergency planning and response are faced with a complex web of prima facie obligations. These obligations can be categorized and a taxonomy of the obligations developed based on how they come into existence. Role obligations are central to professional obligations, but the account of obligations described here provides reasons to rethink the traditional way of conceiving of the PHP's duty to care in situations of public health emergency preparedness and response. The duty of care is a core role obligation that continues to exist, whatever the level of risk or whether or not individuals have consented to be so bound. However, because this duty is a prima facie obligation, it can be overridden legitimately by other obligations, in at least some cases. Several practical issues that have emerged from the published empirical evidence about behavior during actual or potential public health emergency preparedness and response cases suggest that much work can be done in advance to be certain that we are better able to respond to such emergencies. However, the necessary theoretical work must also be done to ensure that PHPs are clearer about the nature of their obligations and thereby better able to fulfill them, even in times of emergency.

Acknowledgments

I would like to thank the participants in the Symposium on Ethics and Public Health Emergency Preparedness and Response held at the Center for the Advancement of Applied Ethics and Political Philosophy, Carnegie Mellon University, Pittsburgh, Pennsylvania, May 4, 2008, for comments on an earlier draft of this chapter. I particularly thank Alex London, Nicole Hassoun, Bruce Jennings, and John D. Arras for helpful comments on that occasion. I also received excellent comments on a later draft from Ross Upshur, Cecile Bensimon, Adrian Viens, and Bruce Jennings. I am very grateful to the Centre for Ethics, University of Toronto, where I completed the penultimate version of this chapter, for funding a Faculty Fellowship for the academic year 2007–08, and to the Joint Centre for Bioethics, University of Toronto, where I completed the final version, for funding a Senior Research Fellowship for the academic year 2008–09.

Notes

1. Moral reasons are, of course, only one type of reason. Just because there is a moral reason for doing something does not mean that we ought to do it (for there may be a more pressing nonmoral reason not to do so, or there may be other more pressing moral reasons to do something else). There are many complicated issues here that go to the heart of contemporary moral theory. See Ridge (2005), Richardson (2007), and Wallace (2008) for discussion of the literature in relation to moral reasons, moral reasoning, and practical reason.

2. For present purposes, we can remain neutral as to what our normative theoretical commitments ought to be. I take "obligation" here to include all of the senses of obligation entailed by, for example, the deontologist's idea of acting from duty, the contractualist's sense of what we owe to each other, as well as the consequentialist's obligation to promote the good. However, once we begin to consider different theoretical commitments, some of the details that follow will also be surprising. See Verweij (2006) for discussion of one such case.

3. Some prefer the phrase "pro tanto" obligations to describe their status. See Richardson (2007). Nothing, here, turns on the phraseology chosen.

4. In this chapter, when I talk of "obligation," I only mean "moral obligation." This is not meant to imply anything about the status of moral obligations in relation to other nonmoral obligations (e.g., legal or prudential obligations). I do not mean to imply that moral obligations cannot be overridden by nonmoral obligations in at least some situations.

5. There are a number of different distinctions that might be used in any attempt to create a priority for certain types of obligations. Here, I discuss just two of the most popular ones: the distinction between agent-neutral and agent-relative reasons and that between perfect and imperfect duties. I will argue that even if such distinctions make sense, they cannot be used to justify giving priority to certain obligations in deliberations about what is appropriate prior to the judgment about what to do in response to a particular situation. Perhaps the most influential philosophical distinction in the contemporary literature that might be used to order sets of obligations is that between agent-relative and agent-neutral reasons (Nagel, 1986, pp. 152–153; Parfit, 1984, p. 184). The distinction is difficult to draw (see Ridge, 2005), but, roughly, agent-relative reasons are those with ineliminable reference to a particular agent, such as my obligations to my family and friends. On this view, *my* agent-relative reasons are distinct from yours because I have special obligations to care for *my* children or *my* parents (in a way that I do not have toward yours). Agent-neutral reasons are considerations that apply to everyone or give everyone reasons to act (e.g., because someone is suffering in pain). One reason that this account has been so influential is that it is used to claim that (at least some forms of) consequentialism (allegedly) have no place for agent-relative obligations, and, because we think there are such obligations, this provides a reason to think that such an approach to moral theory is mistaken (or needs to be supplemented in some way). There is no suggestion, even from those who accept this implicit anti-consequentialism, that this means that agent-relative reasons (of a certain type) are the only relevant obligations or that they should always take priority over the agent-neutral obligations where it is accepted that we have both. However, the latter view is an implication that remains tempting. Such a view would maintain that in a clash between agent-relative and agent-neutral reasons, the former would

have some sort of priority. A frequently used example can be taken to imply this priority as follows: in a clash between a commitment to a member of your own family in need and a general obligation to strangers in need, the former can legitimately take priority (McNaughton & Rawlings, 2007). However, it is important to see that this is a kind of *permission* to take the agent-relative obligation as a priority (in relevant circumstances), not an *ordering* of the two sets of obligations. There is no reason to think in advance of looking at the details of a particular case that the agent-relative will have some sort of precedence. It is easy to imagine situations in which agent-neutral obligations may well take priority. For example, perhaps you have promised to read your child a bedtime story (an agent-relative obligation), but you could alternatively use your time on this one occasion to raise money for charity (an agent-neutral obligation) and thereby save tens of children from starvation. In such a case, it is far from obvious that we should always give priority to the agent-relative obligation. Likewise, it certainly sometimes seems appropriate to be agent-neutral toward all relevant agents (including your own family), such as where you have responsibility for allocating funding from central resources: here, you ought to be impartial and not give priority to those closest to you. Interestingly, Hardimon (1994, pp. 333–334) points out the fact that Nagel (1986) seems to have no real interest in role obligations, and it is not really clear where they fit in his classification.

An alternative way of seeking to make a distinction between types of obligations is the historical division between perfect and imperfect duties. This distinction has a long pedigree in moral philosophy, but many reference the work of Kant (1797/1996) as a key influence on the modern distinction. For Kant, a perfect (or negative) duty is one that prohibits certain actions, and any action that violates such a duty is wrong. An imperfect (or positive) duty is also a pressing requirement, but we have some latitude about when it is appropriate to carry out such duties (1797/1996, pp. 421–424). In medical ethics, the distinction is often illustrated by reference to the obligation to cause no harm (nonmaleficence—a perfect obligation) and an obligation to provide charitable assistance to one in need (beneficence—an imperfect obligation). (See Beauchamp & Childress, 2008, pp. 149–151 and 198–204, for discussion of the nonmaleficence–beneficence distinction.) Again, the danger is that it is assumed that the purpose of the distinction is to mark a priority of perfect over imperfect duties. However, plausible and sympathetic reconstructions of Kant's views, such as that due to

Sullivan (1994, pp. 99–105), provide clear evidence that this is not the case. It is understandable how the priority is often assumed to apply to the perfect duty because it can seem more "pressing." However, for Kant, imperfect duties bind absolutely, exactly in the way perfect ones do. Where there is conflict between a perfect and imperfect duty, there is no automatic priority of one over the other; it is a matter of judgment which one becomes actually binding. In more modern prima facie formulations of deontology, such as that due to Ross (1930) and, more recently, Beauchamp and Childress (2008), this is treated more formally as officially stipulating that there ought to be no ranking of such principles. On this view, latitude (and responsibility) is given to the agent in relation to all duties. I think this is a far more appropriate way to frame our obligations. (As I have argued elsewhere, if principles are genuinely prima facie, there should be no official or unofficial ordering of them prior to moral judgment in response to a particular case; See Gillon, 2003, for one unofficial ordering and Dawson & Garrard, 2006, for a skeptical response.)

6. A related but distinct concern to the two issues of possible prior ordering of obligations discussed in the previous footnote is that of supererogation. It is often claimed that so-called common sense morality will want to preserve a distinction between our ordinary obligations (those things that we ought to do) and actions that are good but go beyond what we are strictly required to do (the supererogatory) (Kagan, 1989; Urmson, 1958). This is a related concern because it might be argued that ordinary obligations should take some sort of priority over any potentially supererogatory actions. This is perhaps the most important of these related issues because some argue that what we sometimes seem to think of as obligations binding health professionals (e.g., performing their job during an epidemic) are actually supererogatory rather than ordinary obligations. This is a complex issue. However, rather than thinking that there is no obligation to go beyond what is required, we should think of this as being a case where other considerations (including other duties) constrain any tendency to be inappropriately heroic. (For example, a firefighter who risks his own life may place some of his colleagues in danger as a result of his "heroic" action.) Accepting a role for the ideal or the supererogatory does not mean that, at times, our all-things-considered obligation will not be very demanding indeed.

7. This important background role of public health is often forgotten. PHPs are entrusted with significant powers (often backed up by the

law) to fulfill this mandate. It is essential that trust is maintained in public health and the work of public health professionals, and the best means of doing so is through such factors as democratic oversight and clear lines of accountability.

8. Such situations may create obligations of reciprocity owed to the professional (*qua* professional). These will be in addition to any other obligations owed to the individual professional *qua* person, citizen, or the like.

9. It might be argued that such relationships are actually constitutive of an individual's identity as a particular person (Sandel, 1982). However, we don't need to accept this metaphysical view to see the importance of social relations and social roles in the evolution of our moral obligations.

10. We can leave to one side whether this class includes nonhuman persons, although at least some of these general obligations may well be owed to some other nonhuman animals.

11. I think we can also remain neutral as to whether we have obligations to our self.

12. The exact boundaries between beneficence and nonmaleficence are disputed (see Beauchamp & Childress, 2008). Some suggest that we can clearly distinguish the two, but I believe that this is far more difficult than is often thought. For example, we might consider ourselves to have the following obligations, but find them difficult to assign to these two categories: an obligation not to infect others, an obligation to prevent harm, an obligation to remove harm, and an obligation to reduce harm. See Dawson (2007) for discussion of this issue.

13. See Scheffler (1997) for discussion.

14. See Malm et al. (2008) for an outline of such a view and University of Toronto Joint Centre for Bioethics Pandemic Ethics Working Group (2008) for a reply.

15. Something along these lines should meet the objections to Hardimon's proposals put forward by Simmons (1996).

16. This is not to say that there might be other reasons to have such obligations. For example, if I derive benefit from local services it may mean that I have an obligation to contribute to their upkeep as public goods (through financial support such as taxation).

17. This is distinct from the objective/subjective obligations as discussed by Zimmerman (2006).

18. My focus in this chapter is primarily on the obligations relevant to the individual actions of PHPs in relation to public health emergency preparedness and response. However, it is also important to think about other groups who will have obligations in the event of such emergencies. These groups will include those with positions of responsibility within government and government agencies. Depending on the person and his or her role, various professional and role obligations will potentially emerge. For example, being a representative of local, state, or federal government working in public health will result in a set of role obligations, perhaps derived ultimately from the general obligation to protect the public from harm. One vital role obligation will be to consider, in advance, some of the potential problems that might arise in relation to public health emergency preparedness and response and consider ways to create the infrastructure so as to be able to adequately respond when needed. This chapter seeks to contribute to such a task.

19. Daniels's discussion (originally published in 1991) is framed in terms of the risk of HIV infection in the performance of routine medical and surgical procedures. I see no reason to think that some version of the same framework could not be used in the context of public health emergency preparedness and response in general, when we are talking about risks involved in pursuing one's core occupational tasks.

20. The "duty to care" and "duty to treat" are, of course, not strictly synonymous. The "duty to treat" is really a particular form or aspect of the "duty to care." I use the "duty to treat" literature here because it raises parallel issues to those in the "duty to care" case. If a health care professional refuses to "treat" a patient, there is no "care." Discussions in relation to public health have to be wider than "treatment" because the focus of much activity is not just treatment but prevention and protection. These latter activities can fall under a "duty of care" (in addition to any "duty to treat"). In my view, it is a mistake to conceptualize the issues around HIV solely in terms of an individualistic "duty to treat" perspective, but that's another story to be saved for a different occasion.

21. This way of framing the issue is the standard view in the literature. See, for example, Arras (1988) and Morin, Higginson, and Goldrich

(2006) for other examples of this approach. Even those who, rightly, in my view, want to broaden out and contextualize the discussion of a duty to care (such as Bensimon, Tracy, Bernstein, Zlotnik Shaul, & Upshur, 2007) seem beholden to this general framework. See, for example, the way that the questions are phrased in the interview guide used by Bensimon et al. (2007, p. 2574).

22. I mean this to be an attempt to become clearer about the status of the relevant obligations. Of course, if an individual "goes beyond" what is required, I do not wish to imply that he or she ought to criticized or condemned.

23. If there is any doubt about this, I suggest the reader asks some members of the public whether they can imagine a doctor or nurse having no such obligation! See also Bensimon et al. (2007) for empirical support for the widespread acceptance of this view.

24. We also need to take care not to be misled in our characterization of the relevant ethical considerations by purely contingent features of the US health care system. The fact that many US physicians choose to see their relationships with patients as purely contractual does not mean that they should do so.

25. Some may object to my use of the language of "failure." However, I think it is important to signal that there can be cases where we fail to do what we ought to do. Such moral failings may carry different amounts of culpability.

26. There is certainly a case for debating and revisiting professional codes so that any obligations are made explicit (University of Toronto Joint Centre for Bioethics Pandemic Influenza Working Group, 2005), and some jurisdictions actually have provisions for conscripting essential staff in the face of a shortage of key personnel.

27. Reid (2006) argues along these lines, suggesting that there is a broad social contract at work behind the duty to care and that we should not think about such a duty as being something that merely binds particular health care professionals. It is unfair to leave individuals to take up the burdens of society's choices and failures.

28. My discussion has focused on health care professionals. The issues may be slightly different with nonprofessional essential staff, such as cleaners, morticians, porters, and the like. We should also think about what issues such groups face and how we can respond to their concerns.

References

Arras, J. D. (1988). The fragile web of responsibility: AIDS and the duty to treat. *Hastings Center Report*, *18*, S10–19.

Beauchamp, T., & Childress, J. (2008). *Principles of biomedical ethics* (6th ed.). Oxford: Oxford University Press.

Bensimon, C. M., Tracy, C. S., Bernstein, M., Zlotnik Shaul, R., & Upshur, R. E. G. (2007). A qualitative study of the duty to care in communicable disease outbreaks. *Social Science and Medicine*, *65*, 2566–2575.

Daniels, N. (2006). Duty to treat or right to refuse? In M. J. Selgelid, M. P. Battin, & C. B. Smith (Eds.), *Ethics and infectious disease*. Oxford: Blackwell, 147–170. [Reprinted from: Daniels, N. (1991). Hastings Center Report, *21*, 2.]

Dawson, A. (2007). Herd protection as a public good: Vaccination and our obligations to others. In A. Dawson & M. Verweij (Eds.), *Ethics, prevention and public health*. Oxford: Oxford University Press, 160–177.

Dawson, A., & Garrard, E. (2006). In defence of moral imperialism: Four equal and universal prima facie duties. *Journal of Medical Ethics*, *32*, 200–204.

Dwyer, J., & Tsai, D. (2008). Developing the duty to treat: HIV, SARS, and the next epidemic. *Journal of Medical Ethics*, *34*, 7–10.

Gillon, R. (2003). Ethics needs principles—Four can encompass the rest—and respect for autonomy should be "first among equals." *Journal of Medical Ethics*, *29*, 307–312.

Hardimon, M. O. (1994). Role obligations. *Journal of Philosophy*, *91*(7), 333–363.

Jeske, D. (2008). *Special obligations*. Stanford Encyclopedia of Philosophy. Available at http://plato.stanford.edu/entries/special-obligations/.

Kagan, S. (1989). *The limits of morality*. Oxford: Oxford University Press.

Kant, I. (1797/1996). The metaphysics of morals. In M. J. Gregor (Ed.), *Practical philosophy: The Cambridge edition of the works of Immanuel Kant*. Cambridge: Cambridge University Press, 353–604.

Malm, H., May, T., Francis, L. P., Omer, S. B., Salmon, D. A., & Hood, R. (2008). Ethics, pandemics and the duty to treat. *American Journal of Bioethics*, *8*, 4–19.

McNaughton, D., & Rawlings, P. (2007). Deontology. In R. Ashcroft, A. Dawson, H. Draper, & J. McMillan (Eds.), *Principles of health care ethics* (2nd ed.). Chichester: Wiley, 66–71.

Morin, K., Higginson, D., & Goldrich, M. (2006). Physician obligation in disaster preparedness and response. *Cambridge Quarterly of Healthcare Ethics, 15*, 417–431.

Nagel, T. (1986). *The view from nowhere*. New York/Oxford: Oxford University Press.

Parfit, D. (1984). *Reasons and persons*. Oxford: Clarendon Press.

Qureshi, K., Gershon, R. R. M., Sherman, M. F., Straub, T., Gebbie, E., McCollum, M., . . . Morse, S. S. (2005). Health care workers' ability and willingness to report to duty during catastrophic disasters. *Journal of Urban Health, 82*, 378–378.

Reid, L. (2006). Diminishing returns? Risk and the duty to care in the SARS epidemic. In M. J. Selgelid, M. P. Battin, & C. B. Smith (Eds.), *Ethics and infectious disease*. Oxford: Blackwell, 171–199.

Richardson, H. S. (2007) *Moral reasoning*. Stanford Encyclopedia of Philosophy. Available at http://plato.stanford.edu/entries/reasoning-moral/.

Ridge, M. (2005). *Reasons for action: Agent-neutral vs. agent-relative*. Stanford Encyclopedia of Philosophy. Available at http://plato.stanford.edu/entries/reasons-agent/.

Ross, W. D. (1930). *The right and the good*. Oxford: Oxford University Press.

Sandel, M. (1982). *Liberalism and the limits of justice*. Cambridge: Cambridge University Press.

Scheffler, S. (1997). Relationships and responsibilities. *Philosophy and Public Affairs, 26*, 189–209.

Simmons, A. J. (1996). External justification and institutional roles. *Journal of Philosophy, 93*, 28–36.

Straus, S. E., Wilson, K., Rambaldini, G., Rath, D., Lin, Y., Gold, W. Y., & Kapral, M. K. (2004). Severe acute respiratory syndrome and its impact on professionalism: Qualitative study of physicians' behaviour during an emerging healthcare crisis. *British Medical Journal, 329*, 83–86.

Sullivan, R. J. (1994). *An introduction to Kant's ethics*. Cambridge: Cambridge University Press.

University of Toronto Joint Centre for Bioethics Pandemic Influenza Working Group. (2005). *Stand on guard for thee: Ethical considerations in preparedness planning for pandemic influenza*. Toronto: Joint Centre for Bioethics.

University of Toronto Joint Centre for Bioethics Pandemic Ethics Working Group. (2008). The duty to care in a pandemic. *American Journal of Bioethics*, *8*, 31–33.

Urmson, J. O. (1958). Saints and heroes. In A. I. Melden (Ed.), *Essays in moral philosophy*. Seattle: University of Washington Press, 198–216.

Verweij, M. (2006). Obligatory precautions against infection. In M. J. Selgelid, M. P. Battin, & C. B. Smith (Eds.), *Ethics and infectious disease*. Oxford: Blackwell Press, 70–82.

Wallace, R. J. (2008). *Practical reason*. Stanford Encyclopedia of Philosophy. Available at http://plato.stanford.edu/entries/practical-reason/.

Zimmerman, M. J. (2006). Is moral obligation objective or subjective? *Utilitas*, *18*, 329–361.

6

Research in a Public Health Crisis

The Integrative Approach to Managing the Moral Tensions

ALEX JOHN LONDON

Introduction

In the face of a public health crisis, the activity of gathering generalizable scientific or statistical information may seem at best an ancillary project, something that should be postponed until the primary and more urgent goal of mitigating the effects of the crisis has been fully accomplished. When time, resources, and personnel are scarce, and when individuals and communities are at their most vulnerable, the imperative to aid may seem to trump the imperative to learn.

However, when communities are faced with novel contagion, contamination, or other health threat, research may provide the only way to form an accurate understanding of the relevant phenomenon and to translate that understanding into effective plans, policies, or interventions. Similarly, when social institutions enact policies, carry out relief efforts, or deploy other interventions in response to a problem, scientific research may be necessary to ascertain whether the response actually improves the state of affairs, as intended, or whether it is ineffectual or even positively harmful. Failing to use appropriate scientific methods to assess interventions and responses, therefore, may impede the capacity of public health institutions to serve their proper social function now, and, if they never act on the imperative to learn, they will not possess the information needed to improve their capacity to aid in the future.

More salient, therefore, than the threshold question of whether research can be justified in the context of a public health emergency is the question of how to determine which kind of research it is ethically permissible to initiate and what the constraints are on how it should be conducted in practice. In this report, I clarify some of the moral tensions that can arise between activities of public health emergency response and public health emergency research. I discuss two prominent approaches to assessing key ethical dimensions of clinical research whose ability to provide meaningful guidance to the resolution of these tensions is hampered by serious shortcomings. Finally, the report outlines a framework for managing these tensions that permits research in this context only if it integrates the interests of community members and research participants in a particular way. This "integrative approach" sets out terms on which important research can be advanced in this context without compromising the status of research participants as the moral and political equals of their compatriots.

Research and the Fundamental Goals of Emergency Response

In this discussion, the terms "public health crisis" and "public health emergency" are used interchangeably. They refer to a state of affairs in which the health of a substantial portion of a community's members is either compromised or in imminent danger because of the inability of existing mechanisms for safeguarding the public's health to cope with an emergent health threat. In such situations, the immediate or proximate threat may emanate from exposure to infectious disease, chemical agents, or other substances that have life-threatening, debilitating, toxic, or other negative effects. People may be exposed to such threats because the health infrastructure of the community has itself been damaged or compromised. In other cases, such threats may overwhelm existing mechanisms for safeguarding the public's health because of their novel character, because of the size, speed, or magnitude of their health effects.

For the present discussion, we can distinguish three distinct but often overlapping phases of public health crisis response. The *planning and preparedness phase* occurs before the onset of a particular public health emergency. The main goals at this stage are to develop, practice, and evaluate the tools, methods, policies, and procedures that can be used to prevent potential public health threats from rising to the status of an emergency situation or that can be used to safeguard the health interests of individuals and communities in an array of emergency situations. This represents the optimal time to carry out clinical and public health research that is necessary to mount an effective response to major public health threats. Unfortunately, it may not be possible to fully address some research questions during this period.

The *public health crisis response phase* occurs when a public health emergency is detected or perceived to be imminent. The fundamental goal of crisis response is to safeguard the basic health interests of individuals in the affected population. "Basic health interests" here are a subset of what will be referred to as "basic interests." Basic interests are a set of interests that all individuals in a community share in being able to function in certain socially basic ways (London, 2003). A kind of functioning is socially basic if it constitutes a building block, or a prerequisite, for the ability to form, revise, and pursue a life plan from among a wide range of alternatives (Rawls, 1982; Sen, 1982). The set of basic interests includes the freedom to develop and exercise one's talents and abilities, including the ability to associate and to speak freely, to move, to be secure in one's person, and to have one's private information kept confidential. It also includes basic social and economic interests, such as the ability to access public spaces and to secure productive employment (Anderson, 1999; Nussbaum, 2000).

Basic health interests relate specifically to the ability to function in ways that are free from sickness, injury, and disease. Having effective access to potable water, safe food, shelter, and sanitation and living in an environment free from toxins, contagion, and other hazards are basic health interests of individuals and communities. In addition, basic health interests encompass broader interests in having effective access to those factors or determinants of health that affect entire populations because of their close connection to important features of the social, political, and physical environment in which those populations live.

The *post-crisis transition phase* often overlaps with the immediate crisis response phase. This phase occurs during the period of transition in which infrastructure is being rebuilt, the environment is being remediated, or social institutions are being reconfigured to safeguard the basic health interests of community members over the long term. It also includes the time during which displaced populations remain in temporary accommodations without being fully integrated back into the social circumstances in which they have effective access to the means of self-support. The primary goal in this period is to ensure that the basic health interests of individuals in the relevant populations are protected and secured during the time of transition.

The US federal regulations governing human subjects research define "research" as "a systematic investigation, including research development, testing and evaluation, designed to develop or contribute to generalizable knowledge" (US Department of Health and Human Services, 2005). The line between research and public health practice is often blurred because effective pursuit of public health requires the use of various scientific and statistical methods (Centers for Disease Control and Prevention [CDC], 1999, 2010). Moreover, these methods are often used to generate information from which generalizations can be drawn about questions such as disease prevalence, routes of transmission, or the merits of various interventions, policies, or programs. Very often, however, the point of gathering this information is to facilitate the process of enhancing the public health of the population from which the information is gathered, not to generate information that will support inferences about questions that range beyond the immediate health needs of that population.

To avoid confusion, therefore, terms like "scientific methods" or "statistical methods" will refer here to techniques that are used to generate information from which inferences can be drawn with increased confidence about the subject phenomenon. Terms like "research" or "research activity" will refer to the use of these methods in service of the fundamental goal of expanding knowledge and understanding of a phenomenon beyond what is necessary to provide effective emergency response in a particular case. In some instances, this understanding is valued in and of itself. But for most health-related research, and for public health research in particular, the intrinsic value of expanded understanding is secondary to the social value that comes from this increase in knowledge as an engine for generating new tools or methods of intervention; improving future practice, policy, or response; or opening avenues for further inquiry that will produce such results.

It can be difficult to determine when the use of scientific methods crosses from a routine component of public health practice to the conduct of public health research (MacQueen & Huehler, 2004). In the present inquiry, the concern is less with trying to provide a precise demarcation between research and practice than with delineating tensions that can arise between these activities. The fundamental ethical issues in this context grow out of these tensions and how they might be mitigated or resolved. No taxonomy will eliminate ambiguous cases, and the project of crafting a more precise set of regulatory definitions is beyond the scope of this chapter.

Tensions can arise between the activities of public health emergency response and public health research on at least two levels. The first occurs at the level of fundamental goals. Most research activities are concerned with research participants only insofar as they represent data points, the aggregation of which will generate valuable information. This is not a comment about the sympathy, empathy, or good will of researchers, or about the moral character of the research enterprise, but about research insofar as it is a kind of scientific inquiry in which the fundamental goal is to gather data from which relevant inferences can be drawn. The point is simply that in the context of research involving human subjects, the requisite data must be gathered from populations of persons. The potential for conflict arises from the fact that what is required by sound scientific design to generate data that can support the desired inferences and choices relating to who receives which interventions or tests or how various measurements or observations should be carried out may not correspond to what is required to meet the present needs of affected persons or populations.

The criteria for success in the research enterprise, therefore, differ from the criteria for success in emergency response. The success of a research activity is a function of the soundness of its methods, the quality of the data that they generate, and their relevance to future projects. The success of emergency response efforts is a function of the extent to which they succeed in protecting or advancing the basic health interests of affected individuals and communities. These differences in fundamental goals do not imply that these activities cannot be carried out successfully at the same time and in the same context. The point is, rather, that if this is to occur, it must be the result of careful planning and execution. It should also be noted that when it is not possible to reconcile these goals in practice, decisions will have to be made about which set of ends should be subordinated to the other.

This chapter is not concerned with the use of scientific methods that are necessary to properly address a particular public health crisis. When epidemiologic studies, needs assessments, disease surveillance, and other common public health activities are carried out in the service of responding effectively to a public health crisis or threat, they would not constitute research activities for the purpose of this chapter. This does not mean that such activities do not pose risks to the interests of the population under study. Rather, it means that these risks should be minimized and evaluated as reasonable or unreasonable in light of their relationship to the goals of providing effective crisis relief in the particular case. Risks that are not necessary to the provision of effective crisis relief should be eliminated or reduced as far as possible.

Activities constitute research, for the purpose of this discussion, when they employ scientific and statistical methods in ways that diverge from what is necessary to provide effective crisis response in the particular case. They might diverge from this goal by gathering more information than is necessary to provide effective crisis response or by gathering information that does not contribute directly to the provision of emergency response in the particular situation. As a general rule, the extent to which an activity involves a research component can be determined by considering the extent to which its design and execution are primarily determined by the goal of effectuating relief efforts in the particular situation or by the goal of generating information that diverges from this end.

A second tension concerns the potential for conflict in resource allocation. Because research activities and emergency response activities might require different procedures to accomplish their respective ends, they can make competing demands on time, personnel, and other social and economic resources. When such resources are scarce, this tension can create a practical conflict that would require that these activities be prioritized so that resources can be directed only to the most essential or pressing objectives.

For example, personnel from Centers for Disease Control and Prevention (CDC) might be tasked to assist state and local public health entities in evacuating and caring for individuals who are displaced from their homes by flooding. In the course of this deployment, these personnel may encounter an opportunity to study the effectiveness of a brief session of cognitive-behavioral therapy to stabilize the affect of persons who are identified as at risk for a range of mental health problems associated with the stress and anxiety of being displaced. At a general level, the goals of this study diverge from the goals of effective crisis response to the extent that the purpose of the study is to evaluate the merits of a particular mental health intervention. However, this divergence does not necessarily create a practical conflict because it may be possible to conduct this study in a way that actually advances important goals of crisis response.

However, even if it is possible in principle to carry out this research in a way that would advance the goals of emergency response, scarcity of resources can create a conflict in resource allocation that might require that these activities be prioritized appropriately. If sufficient CDC personnel are not available to coordinate the evacuation and care of the affected population *and* carry out this study, these activities would have to be prioritized and the time and energy of trained personnel redirected accordingly.

Current Frameworks for Managing Tensions

An acceptable ethical framework for evaluating research in the public health emergency context should provide practical guidance about how to reconcile the tensions described in the previous section. This practical guidance should also be grounded in a normative foundation that is capable of winning the support of community members who embrace widely divergent life plans and frameworks of value. Unfortunately, the two most common frameworks for assessing the ethical dimensions of clinical research have significant limitations, either in their own right or in the context of research in a public health emergency in particular.

One widely accepted framework for evaluating the ethics of research initiatives relies on the concept of *equipoise*. Developed by the philosopher Charles Fried, the concept of equipoise was given its canonical formulation by Benjamin Freedman (Freedman, 1987, 1990; Fried, 1974). According to Freedman, equipoise exists when there is significant uncertainty in the expert medical community about the relative therapeutic merits of a set of interventions for a particular medical condition. This concept has exerted tremendous influence in the context of research ethics because it holds that when the expert medical community is in equipoise between certain specified interventions, it is morally permissible to allow a patient to be randomized to interventions in that set. This is permissible because allowing the patient's care to be determined by a random process when equipoise exists does not violate what has been referred to as the clinician's "therapeutic obligation" (Marquis, 1983), "duty of personal care" (Fried, 1974), or "fiduciary duty" (Miller & Weijer, 2003) to the individual patient.

This approach has at least three notable virtues (Evans & London, 2006; London, 2007*a*). First, it provides a way of specifying how clinical research can satisfy the requirement that to be acceptable it should have sufficient social value to justify the research. For equipoise to exist, there must be a lack of consensus in the expert medical community about how best to advance the interests of a particular patient population. Trials that are designed to disturb equipoise have social value in that they provide the information that the community needs to resolve such disagreements and, ultimately, to advance the standard of care that is available to patients.

Second, the concept of equipoise provides a way of specifying the general requirement that acceptable research must have a favorable risk–benefit ratio. It does this by using the physician's duty of personal care to set the bound on acceptable risk in the research context. Risks are reasonable, in this view, when they are consistent with the clinician's duty to meet the needs of each individual patient to the best of his or her ability.

Finally, this approach specifies these moral requirements in a way that is operationally useful. That is, it provides practical guidance for making decisions about clinical research in a way that goes beyond the raw intuitions of deliberators.

This approach has been subject to intense scrutiny since its inception, and recently this criticism has intensified (Gifford, 1986, 1995, 2000; Hellman, 2002; Miller & Brody, 2003). I illustrate here one major problem in trying to apply this approach to the context of emergency public health research. Its moral foundation is built on a duty that individual clinicians owe to their individual patients. In the context of public health, however, the personnel carrying out research may not be physicians, and participants are not patients but are populations or communities. Similarly, public health research will often involve participants who are healthy but who face a range of risks to their health from a variety of social, environmental, physical, psychological, chemical, or biological threats. It is questionable, therefore, whether the duty of personal care that physicians owe to patients is the proper model for the obligations that nonphysician researchers owe to healthy participants in communities in public health research.

Moreover, certain forms of public health research might have the potential to have a substantial impact on the interests of community members even though they do not directly recruit or enroll individual participants and then allocate them to different arms or conditions, as is done in clinical trials. Rather, public health research might study alternative methods of restoring access to rudimentary building blocks of the public's health, such as removing a toxin from the environment or restoring access to potable water in the aftermath of a natural disaster or terror attack. In such cases, the relevant interventions might be carried out by engineers, and different interventions might be randomized to sets of affected areas. Such research might have an impact on the interests of members of the affected community, but it is difficult to see why this research should be constrained by the obligations of physicians, as opposed to some other set of social obligations.

Concerns about the applicability of the normative foundation of this view are amplified by the fact that there is a long tradition in public health of making the health of the public the primary moral focus of the profession. As a result, even when public health researchers are physicians, they face an ethical question about whether their activities should be bounded by the moral norms of clinical medicine rather than by some more social ethic. A simple appeal to the obligations of the physician is not sufficient to answer the operative social question of which set of norms should govern the activities of medical professionals who are charged with advancing public rather than individual health.

The second major framework for evaluating the ethics of research initiatives, the duty not to exploit persons (Miller & Brody, 2003), does not appeal to the duties of physicians to specify fundamental moral requirements. Because the proponents of this approach take the duty not to exploit to be somewhat weaker than the physician's duty of personal care, this approach allows subjects to be offered risks that would be unacceptable in the former model. Because this approach does not rely on the duties of clinicians for its operational content, it can also be ported into the public health context more readily.

The primary drawback of this approach, however, is that it leaves the content of key requirements largely unspecified (London, 2006*a*, 2007*a*, 2007*b*). For example, one way a study can be exploitative is if its anticipated benefits do not outweigh its attendant risks. As in the Common Rule, the benefits in question here are not limited to those that might accrue to research participants (US Department of Health and Human Services, 2005). Risks to participants can be justified solely by benefits to society. In this framework, it is clear that the interests of individual research participants can be compromised as long as the research is in service of sufficient social good. It is not clear, however, how to conceive of the social good in a way that might assist decision-makers in making the relevant tradeoffs. That is, are the risks to trial participants supposed to be weighed against the number of potential lives saved in the future from the results of a particular trial; the social utility of the information a trial generates; some other metric, such as dollars; or some complex mixture of such options? Even if decision-makers believe that they can specify the relevant social utilities, they still need to know how to trade those utilities against the risks to individual research participants. How much social value needs to be generated to offset the prospect of a serious adverse event for one participant?

As Aristotle wisely cautioned, more precision should not be demanded from an ethical framework than the subject matter permits. However, this is likely to be an area where the intuitions of reasonable people differ and in which stakeholders will require operationally meaningful guidance in order to move beyond conflicting intuitions. The problem with the unvarnished injunction to ensure a reasonable ratio of benefits and burdens is not that there is no way to make such an assessment. It is that the various ways to carry out such an assessment are limited only by the imaginations of different individuals.

This is of special concern in the context of public health because its community-focused disciplinary perspective dovetails naturally with a utilitarian approach to resolving the tensions outlined previously. Utilitarianism is a foundational moral theory that holds that the only factor relevant to determining the rightness of conduct is the goodness of the state of affairs that it produces. Classical utilitarian theories focus on conduct at the level of individual actions and hold that, in each particular case, agents are obligated to choose the act that maximizes the aggregate social welfare.

A utilitarian approach to evaluating the risks and benefits of clinical research has a certain appeal for several reasons. First, it appears to provide a clear decision procedure for evaluating risks. Risks to the welfare of research participants are summed and then compared with the potential for increased welfare that the trial offers to future beneficiaries of its results. Second, it makes this evaluation from a social standpoint, according to which each individual is regarded as the equal of every other. More precisely, each unit of a person's welfare is given the same weight when welfare scores are summed together. Finally, even those who reject utilitarian approaches to social problems under ordinary circumstances may view public health emergencies as extraordinary circumstances. In the face of a pandemic, for example, utilitarianism's focus on maximizing aggregate welfare might be seen as a particular virtue.

However, such an appeal to utilitarianism suffers from a range of problems, only two of which will be mentioned here. First, this approach tramples on what is referred to as the *separateness of persons* (Rawls, 1971); that is, utilitarianism treats everyone equally in the sense that it gives equal weight to each unit of utility, no matter whose utility it is. As a result, utilitarianism does not regard individual agents as morally special. Rather, each unit of utility is treated as an input into what is morally special, namely, the total utility of the social aggregate. If the latter can be increased by compromising the rights or welfare of a few, then decision-makers are required, not simply permitted, to do to those individuals whatever it takes to ensure the greatest social utility.

This has profound practical implications because the benefits received by the aggregate can easily overwhelm harms to research participants. For instance, if enough people stand to benefit from the results of a study, it may be permissible to allow even a fairly sizable population of research participants to suffer severe, preventable harms, including death. Moreover, if each unit of welfare is given the same weight, regardless of whose welfare it is, then sacrificing the health and welfare of participants would be permissible in research that aims to produce even the most optional social luxuries as long as those benefits are enjoyed by enough future beneficiaries. Because the time horizon of the future is so vast, this will almost always be the case.

Those who are sympathetic to utilitarianism have proposed a variety of responses to such objections. One important response is, perhaps somewhat paradoxically, to claim that even the classical utilitarian would reject such an approach to conducting clinical trials because such crude efforts to maximize social welfare would ultimately fail. In particular, whereas this approach may sound good from the comfort of one's armchair, even the perception that social institutions are permitted to sacrifice the basic health interests of some in order to promote the welfare of others would have profoundly corrosive effects on public trust. Not only would it make it extremely difficult to recruit research participants, it would impede the willingness of community members to cooperate with public health institutions when individuals are at their most vulnerable and when the support of those institutions is needed the most.

These worries are far from theoretical. The legacy of the now infamous Tuskegee syphilis study appears to continue to play a role in an undercurrent of distrust of public health in general and public health research in particular in African American communities (Freimuth et al., 2001; McCallum, Arekere, Green, Katz, & Rivers, 2006). In fact, postal workers referenced this study when expressing their distrust of public health interventions and research that were carried out in the wake of the 2001 anthrax attacks in the United States (Blanchard et al., 2005; Quinn, Thomas, & McAllister,

2005). The potential for the actions of public health officials to create public distrust and for that distrust to impede the pursuit of major public health goals was stressed by the Working Group on "Governance Dilemmas" in Bioterrorism Response, when they noted that social trust is often confounded by conditions that are typical of public health emergencies such as disease or widespread fear of it and the associated stress that such emergencies place on existing social and economic divisions within a community (Working Group on "Governance Dilemmas" in Bioterrorism Response, 2004). They emphasized that, in such a context, the actions of officials or representatives of major social institutions have a profound influence on the way that the public will respond to subsequent instructions and imperatives.

Some utilitarians have therefore argued that the proper corrective to such problems is not to modify the theory but to take account of all the potential consequences of permitting certain tradeoffs in clinical research. That is, it is not sufficient to compare the risks to subjects against benefits to future beneficiaries. Decision-makers must also consider all the social effects of such a choice, including the social impact that such a decision will have on things like the willingness of others to trust, support, and cooperate with basic social institutions. As a result, they must evaluate a much more expansive set of variables, including how one's present choice may influence the decisions and conduct of others in the future and what the likely consequences of such future choices will be.

Although this may attenuate some of the more objectionable features of classical utilitarianism, it vastly increases the complexity and difficulty of the calculations that must be made to evaluate a particular decision. In fact, it becomes unclear how real decision-makers could even gather all the information that would be necessary to set up this decision problem let alone find the optimal solution to it. Plausibility, therefore, must be purchased at the price of simplicity and parsimony.

To reintroduce simplicity and parsimony, utilitarians may opt to change their focus from evaluating the consequences of individual choices to evaluating the consequences of adopting a set of social rules or policies. Given the corrosive effects of perceived breaches of the public's trust on both public health research and practice, such a rule-utilitarian approach would likely prohibit practices in which the basic interests of research participants are knowingly and avoidably compromised for the benefit of future populations. For the rule utilitarian, then, policies that respect the basic interests of research participants might have the best long-term consequences, even if this means that some individual studies are not as informative as they might be.

Those who reject the equipoise requirement have sometimes characterized their approach as explicitly utilitarian (Miller & Brody, 2007). These comments illustrate one way in which the universe of utilitarian theories is itself quite diverse. Rule utilitarianism is only one variant among many, and different utilitarian theories may diverge in their practical recommendations. These comments also illustrate that, without better guidance about what kind of utilitarian approach should be used to guide decision-making, this alternative effectively leaves deliberators free to adopt, explicitly or implicitly, a diverse range of standards that can lead to widely divergent moral assessments.

The Integrative Approach to Research in the Public Health Emergency Context

To fulfill the social mission of providing practical guidance to decision-makers who embrace diverse and divergent life plans, an adequate framework for evaluating research should have at least three features. First, it should articulate a normative foundation that is suitable for regulating public health research. Second, real decision-makers should be able to gather the information necessary to set up what that framework holds as the relevant decision problem. Finally, it should provide operational guidance about the standards that need to be met in order for research to be permissible in this context.

The integrative approach, which has been described elsewhere (London, 2006*a*, 2007*b*), has the advantage of using a very general normative foundation to derive the kind of operationally meaningful guidance regarding the ethical conduct of research that is the hallmark of approaches that embrace the equipoise requirement. Because its normative foundation is more general in scope, however, this approach applies to a much wider range of cases than do frameworks that draw their normative force from the duties of physicians. It also provides clearer operational guidance than approaches that reject the equipoise requirement. After outlining the normative foundation of the integrative approach, this chapter formulates some of its key principles in a way that applies directly to the context of public health emergency research.

The integrative approach begins with the recognition that, in liberal democratic communities, individuals may differ radically in their personal interests, and these differences are a common source of conflict in social decision-making and public policy. This has implications for research ethics in that a diverse community is likely to disagree about fundamental issues such as the importance of answering certain questions, the significance of whatever risks may be involved in doing so, and how those risks should be traded against the prospect of advances in knowledge.

To facilitate a decision-making process that can secure the support of stakeholders in this context, the integrative approach articulates a social position of common ground from which decisions can be made about how basic social institutions should be regulated, and it defines a particular "space of equality" that delineates the domain over which community members have a just claim to equal treatment. It does so by building on a distinction first drawn by John Rawls, who argued that the first-order conflict over values and ends that predominates pluralistic, liberal communities is predicated on a shared, higher order interest of each individual in being able to advance his or her first-order interests effectively without unwarranted outside interference (Rawls, 1982).

Although individuals may adopt particular life plans that have little in common or that conflict or diverge in fundamental ways, each can recognize that all require the ability to cultivate and to exercise certain basic physical, intellectual, emotional, and social capacities in order to be able to pursue a life plan. Moreover, despite differences in dress, demeanor, or aspiration, each can recognize every other as their moral and political equal in the following respect: their ability to pursue a distinctive and meaningful life plan is predicated on their ability to safeguard and advance these basic interests. As a result, the higher order interest that individuals in diverse and pluralistic communities share in being able to advance their individual life plans provides a ground for giving special evaluative significance to the interest that those individuals have in being able to cultivate the basic intellectual, emotional, physical, and social capacities that make it possible to pursue such a life plan.

The integrative approach thus holds that the basic institutions of a society treat individuals as political equals not by striving to advance the particular ends of any set of individuals, but by safeguarding and advancing, for each individual, those basic interests that make possible the pursuit of a reasonable life plan from among a rich array of possible alternatives. That is, these basic institutions operate in a way that is fair by working to ensure that every individual can function effectively in those rudimentary ways that are necessary to be able to pursue some distinctive life plan. In this regard, the integrative approach seeks to be more responsive to the separateness of persons by laying out terms on which the basic structures of a community can respect the status of each community member as the political equal of every other without summing the interests of community members together.

The integrative approach uses this focus on basic interests for three closely related purposes. First, it provides both a moral and a political ground for a claim to assistance from their compatriots on the part of those whose basic interests are threatened, endangered, or inadequately protected. In particular, the integrative approach holds that when the basic interests of some are threatened by a public health emergency, each has an equal claim on the basic institutions of his or her society to use the best practices available to safeguard and to advance his or her basic health interests.

Second, the imperative to meet these claims as effectively and efficiently as possible provides the justification for creating a social division of labor in which some community members are empowered to advance the basic interests of others in a particular sphere or domain. The institutions that are charged with safeguarding and advancing public health represent one element in such a social division of labor. These institutions are granted special powers and prerogatives that enable them to carry out such duties more effectively. In this way, an institutional framework is created in which those who are willing to take on, as part of their particular life plan, the project of preserving the basic health interests of community members are empowered to do so in a way that benefits everyone.

Finally, this focus on basic interests provides both a moral target for research and a moral constraint on the way that it is carried out. The moral target of research is established by focusing on the link between the basic interests of community members and the network of social institutions that are necessary to preserve and advance them. To improve the capacity of these institutions to fulfill their social role more effectively in the future, community members have a compelling interest in supporting research that will bridge the gap between the basic health needs of community members and the capacity of the health-related institutions in that community to meet those needs (London, 2005). The integrative approach thus grounds a strong social imperative to carry out public health research that is necessary to provide more effective methods or interventions for responding to pressing, future public health threats. It also provides support, under appropriate conditions, for permitting research on phenomena that emerge primarily in the context of a public health crisis, where there is significant social value to improving understanding of these phenomena and where the necessary information could not be collected in a non-crisis context.

This focus on basic interests also grounds the constraints that are placed on the operation of basic social institutions in general and the conduct of public health research in particular. The integrative approach holds that such institutional frameworks must themselves be arranged so as to respect the basic interests of the individuals whose efforts they are designed to coordinate and shape. Whereas those whose basic interests are threatened or endangered in some way can make a legitimate claim on their compatriots to provide them with aid or relief, no party can claim that the preservation or advancement of their basic interests is more important than the basic interests of their compatriots. As a result, all that anyone can claim of their compatriots is a duty to forge an institutional framework that creates opportunities for community members to participate in research that will advance science for the common good without compromising the status of research participants as the political equals of their compatriots in the process. That is, they can legitimately ask their compatriots to dedicate their time and energy and to accept some personal risk in order to facilitate important public health research, but they cannot ask their compatriots to sacrifice their basic interests in the process.

This perspective is partly expressed in the principle of *equality* (see Box 6.1).

Unlike the norms of the physician–patient relationship, the principle of equality has a broad scope of application for two reasons. First, it is grounded in a general moral duty that individuals owe to one another, regardless of their social role, because the basic interests of individuals are intimately bound up with their capacity

BOX 6.1 Principle of Equality

As a necessary condition for ethical permissibility, research with human subjects must be designed and carried out so as not to undermine the standing of research participants as the moral and political equals of their compatriots, either by knowingly compromising their basic interests or by showing unequal concern for their basic interests and those whose interests the research is intended to serve.

for individual agency and welfare, and all persons have a general duty to respect the welfare and autonomy of persons. Second, and perhaps more importantly, the integrative approach derives this principle from a purely political approach to the question of how to organize the basic institutions of a community so that they can be justified as fundamentally fair to those whose rights, liberty, and welfare they affect. This gives the integrative approach an immediate relevance to public health research that the equipoise requirement lacks because of the latter's reliance on the parochial, role-related norms of the physician–patient relationship.

Making the Integrative Approach Operational: Conflicts in Goals

To specify the terms on which relevant research can be advanced without compromising the status of research participants as the moral and political equals of their compatriots, the integrative approach adopts the following two operational criteria (Box 6.2).

Condition A denotes that it is never acceptable to expose research participants to risks that are gratuitous or higher than is necessary (Emanuel, Wendler, & Grady, 2000; US Department of Health and Human Services, 2005). The rationale for conducting research during a public health emergency should relate to the importance of the knowledge that will be generated, either for addressing the immediate crisis or for understanding phenomena, dynamics, or conditions that cannot be feasibly studied in another context. This requirement also covers more than risks to basic interests because research participants can have interests that are of great personal importance even though they are not widely shared and do not constitute a building block needed to function in socially rudimentary ways.

Condition B articulates the mechanism that determines the level of care and protection that must be provided to research participants to ensure that they are respected as the moral equals of their compatriots. It does this by allowing participants to be allocated only to trial arms that provide a level of care or protection

BOX 6.2 First Operational Criterion for Preserving Equality

A necessary condition for ethically acceptable research in the context of a public health emergency is that (A) the risks to subjects should be reduced to those that are necessary to address an important public health question; and (B) when their basic interests are threatened by sickness, injury, or disease, research participants must receive a level of care and protection for their basic interests that does not fall below what at least a reasonable minority of the expert public health community would regard as the most appropriate method of crisis response available.

that does not fall below what at least a reasonable minority of the expert public health community would recommend as the method with the best overall prospect of safeguarding or advancing their basic interests. The focus on not falling below this standard is meant to convey that even when there is a high level of uncertainty or widespread disagreement about what constitutes the best response to a particular problem, it is often possible to identify interventions that would not be advocated as the best response to that problem by even a reasonable minority of the relevant expert community (Kadane, 1996).

In contrast to condition A, condition B focuses on the basic interests of research participants. Two points should be made about this. First, although the agencies that are charged with protecting different aspects of the public's health are primarily concerned with safeguarding and advancing the basic health interests of people, research may pose risks to participants that reach beyond their basic health interests. For example, if sensitive personal information about individuals is recorded in a way that can be linked back to those parties, disclosure of this information may jeopardize their ability to maintain certain personal relationships, their career, or their social standing. Those who conduct such research, therefore, have a duty to keep this information confidential in order to protect the basic interests of research participants. Guideline 18 of the Council for International Organizations of Medical Sciences International Ethical Guidelines for Biomedical Research Involving Human Subjects states that "The investigator must establish secure safeguards of the confidentiality of subjects' research data. Subjects should be told the limits, legal or other, to the investigators' ability to safeguard confidentiality and the possible consequences of breaches of confidentiality." The duty to preserve confidentiality is not absolute, however, and researchers may be under ethical or legal obligation to report certain information that bears directly on public health interests (Council for International Organizations of Medical Sciences, 2002).

Second, condition B articulates the limitations on what kind of offers researchers can make to potential research participants whose interests are threatened in a public health emergency. The focus on basic interests in this condition reflects the idea that community members owe one another a social division of labor that preserves and protects the rudimentary building blocks that individuals need in order to be free to pursue a distinctive life plan. To preserve trust in the social institutions of research and public health, and to preserve their commitment to giving equal regard to the basic interests of each community member, it is not permissible to offer to those whose interests are threatened by a public health emergency participation in studies that provide a lower level of care and protection for the participants' basic interests. However, community members can ask one another to risk, sacrifice, alter, or limit in some way ends or goals that are part of their individual life plan in an effort to secure for others the freedom to pursue and revise such a life plan of their own. In this view, properly functioning institutional review boards should permit public health researchers to ask participants to endure unpleasant experiences or inconveniences or to bear other burdens that do not compromise their basic interests, so long as such risks or burdens are necessary for the conduct of sound science and have been reduced as far as possible. It is then up to individuals, through the process of informed consent, to evaluate these offers and to decide whether those particular burdens are reasonable in light of the goals of the research.

Additional guidance beyond what is contained in condition B is necessary for two reasons. First, the conduct of research may require additional tests or procedures that are necessary to gather sufficient information but might not be conducted if research was not being carried out. The immediate effects of such procedures often implicate the personal interests of individuals in that they involve discomfort or some degree of bodily or personal intrusion. Even when this is the case, such procedures also pose some incremental risk to the basic interests of research participants. In such situations, additional guidance is necessary to determine when such incremental risks to the basic interests of participants are consistent with an equal regard for the basic interests of participants and nonparticipants.

Second, not all research that might be proposed in this context would evaluate methods of crisis intervention or response. It might be desirable to conduct such research in populations where it is not yet necessary to deploy emergency response interventions or in populations where such measures have already been successful deployed.

To deal with risks that arise from purely research-related elements of such research, the integrative approach adopts a second operational criterion (Box 6.3).

The second operational criterion embodies the recognition that, in pursuing their particular projects and goals, individuals routinely assume some degree of risk to their basic interests. Respecting the moral equality of individuals, therefore, cannot require that they be prohibited from voluntarily assuming some degree of risk to their basic interests because such a standard simply could not be achieved. For the integrative approach, the challenge is to establish when incremental risks to the basic interests of individuals violate the underlying commitment to moral equality.

BOX 6.3 Second Operational Criterion for Preserving Equality

In all cases, the cumulative incremental risks to the basic interests of individuals that are derived from research activities that are not offset by the prospect of direct benefit to the individual must not be greater than the risks to the basic interests of individuals that are permitted in the context of other socially sanctioned activities that are similar in structure to the research enterprise.

To increase the practical applicability of these operational criteria, their content must be refined (London, 2006*a*, 2007*b*). This can be done in the context of public health emergency response by considering two broad classes of research. The first is public health research that is directly targeted at evaluating or developing methods or interventions for public health emergency response in populations whose interests are at risk. This class of research has special importance because of its direct relevance to the capacity of public health institutions to fulfill their social role more effectively in the future. The second is public health research on phenomena that emerge primarily in the context of a public health crisis, where the relevant information could not be generated in a non-crisis context.

The integrative approach uses the following test to apply the first operational criterion in practice. This test is used to evaluate research in the first category (Box 6.4).

This test ensures that two important objectives are met. First, it articulates the conditions that decision-makers can use to determine whether participants in a particular trial receive a level of care or relief that does not fall below what would be recommended as the most appropriate method for providing emergency response by at least a reasonable minority of experts in public health (Kadane, 1996). It does this by permitting individuals to be allocated to

BOX 6.4 Practical Test for the First Operational Criterion

When evaluating one or more methods or interventions for public health emergency response, individuals must be allocated only to methods or interventions about which there is either conflict between or uncertainty among the expert public health community about whether the basic health interests of individuals could be more adequately safeguarded or advanced by the provision of methods other than those under study, all things considered.

interventions on the condition of either uncertainty or conflict about the relative merits of those interventions or methods in the particular case.

Uncertainty in this context refers to a state in which relevant public health experts have not formed a settled opinion about whether one mode of crisis response is superior to another. This is not a state of indifference, which I consider a belief that the methods in question are of equivalent value. Uncertainty, in contrast, represents the state in which the evidence supporting the relative merits of candidate interventions is not of sufficient quantity or quality to ground the inference that one is better than the relevant comparator. The determination of the relevant comparator depends on the state of knowledge in the relevant expert community. If, for instance, there is no known effective intervention for a condition, then a no-treatment or placebo arm may be an appropriate comparator. If there are several known effective interventions, one or more of these may be the appropriate comparator, or the investigational agent may be compared to a placebo that is administered in addition to standard treatment. In all cases, the role of research is to generate the information that will allow experts to clarify the relative merits of the various options in an effort to narrow the zone of uncertainty or conflict and to forge a social consensus on the appropriate standard of care.

In the initial phases of the severe acute respiratory syndrome (SARS) outbreak, for example, personnel in some locations chose to provide only supportive care to those believed to have been infected, whereas personnel in other areas moved more quickly to provide therapeutic interventions that would cover a wide range of bacterial and viral pathogens (Muller, McGeer, Straus, Hawryluck, & Gold, 2004). During this time, ribavirin was identified as a promising therapeutic agent, although considerable uncertainty remained about the relative balance of risks and benefits associated with this treatment. The existence of this uncertainty led investigators to attempt to design a clinical trial to evaluate the efficacy of ribavirin. However, the isolation of SARS coronavirus (SARS-CoV) and the in vitro susceptibility studies that this made possible, along with increasing reports of toxicity associated with that drug, were sufficient to bring personnel in Toronto to discontinue ribavirin as a treatment for SARS.

There is no consensus on the best practice for treating SARS (Stockman, Bellamy, & Garner, 2006). However, if new animal and in vitro studies and increased understanding of SARS-CoV had led experts in some communities to favor one set of interventions, while experts in other communities began to favor a different set, the expert clinical community would have moved from a state of uncertainty into a state of conflict.

In contrast to uncertainty, *conflict* refers to the state of affairs in which at least a reasonable minority of experts champion one method as superior to some other method for providing disaster relief in a particular situation while at least a reasonable minority of other experts champions another method as superior to the former. In this case, each side has a determinate conviction about what is best for members of the affected population. If those convictions cannot be jointly satisfied, then they are in conflict (Levi, 1986). The integrative approach permits individuals to be allocated—at random or by some other appropriate method—to any intervention that would be recommended for them by at least a reasonable minority of public health experts.

The integrative approach thus differs from versions of the equipoise requirement that require individual experts to be uncertain. In the most extreme case of conflict, no individual expert is personally uncertain. Each has a definitive preference. The problem is that the preferences of different experts conflict. In this case, the integrative approach permits participants to be allocated to any intervention that would be recommended for them by at least a reasonable minority of public health experts. Versions of the equipoise requirement that require individual experts to be uncertain would not permit research to go forward under such conditions. However, prohibiting research in the face of conflict does nothing to settle the substantive disagreement in the field over the relative merits of the competing interventions. It merely consigns the affected populations to receive a particular intervention—perhaps as a result of the contingent fact about who gets to make the relevant decision—without using the research methods necessary to settle the substantive issue about whether one of the alternatives is better than the others (Evans & London, 2006).

This highlights the second important feature of the first practical test. Namely, it promotes research that has significant social value. This social value emanates from the fact that research that meets this test is designed to resolve substantive conflicts about best practices and, thereby, to advance the capacity of social institutions to provide more effective emergency response in the future.

It might be objected that public health emergencies can be rapidly evolving situations in which information is sparse and not uniformly reliable. When pathogens are novel, the information base might be insufficient to support either adequate clinical or public health responses or useful research. In this context, public health personnel might have to engage in a more informal process of learning through trial and error. Such a process, the objection holds, would not fit neatly into the evaluative framework articulated here.

This objection points to a kind of inquiry that may be necessary to deal with a novel emerging public health threat. This will be referred to as the *abductive phase of inquiry*, in which the term "abduction" refers to the process of generating hypotheses that could then be attractive candidates for testing in a formal research project.

In nonemergency situations, the standard paradigm for facilitating scientific progress is to conduct as much abductive work as possible in settings that do not involve human subjects. That is, basic science, in vitro research, and research with nonhumans are designed to create a model of the condition in question, identify potential interventions, and determine whether there is enough evidence for the therapeutic, prophylactic, or diagnostic promise of candidate interventions to permit their introduction into humans. This division of labor also represents the best way to prepare for a public health crisis. The sudden emergence of a novel threat, however, may require, not that this process be abandoned, but that it be modified to provide to humans interventions whose therapeutic, diagnostic, or prophylactic merits have not yet been validated.

Previous accounts of the information that will need to be gathered to lay the groundwork for successful research in a public health crisis include descriptions of those areas that might require abductive work. Such work includes clarifying the selection criteria for determining the relevant treatment population, defining an intervention or set of interventions that represents the most attractive candidates for clinical use, selecting a hypothesis that it is feasible to test and whose resolution will have significant clinical value, and defining informative and feasible study outcomes (Muller et al., 2004). Although abductive work does not fit neatly into the standard categories of treatment or research, its conduct can still be guided by the framework set out here.

Abductive work has some affinities with clinical or public health practice to the extent that it involves performing tests or deploying interventions in an effort to help a particular population. But it deviates from the paradigm of standard clinical or public health practice to the extent that it involves deploying interventions of unknown efficacy. This might be described by saying that there is a therapeutic aspiration that is shared with standard practices of public health emergency response, but there is a major difference in the lack of the usual degree of justification or scientific support for the proposition that the intervention is likely to achieve the desired goal.

Abductive work also has affinities with clinical or public health research to the extent that interventions are deployed in order to learn about variables, such as the characteristics of the pathogen in question, its responsiveness to certain challenges, and which modalities of intervention might have the most therapeutic, prophylactic, or diagnostic merit. However, it does not fit neatly into the traditional clinical or public health research paradigm because its goal is not to test a hypothesis about the merits of a set of specific interventions but to find hypotheses that are worth testing.

A virtue of the framework outlined here is that it is grounded in a normative foundation that is sufficiently general to apply across a variety of settings. It is worth highlighting three requirements that this framework imposes on abductive activities. First, this is an integrative approach because it tries to find ways of resolving social conflicts that safeguard and advance the underlying basic interests of the relevant parties. In this case, disaster victims have an interest in having their basic health interests protected or advanced, and the broader community has an interest in generating the knowledge necessary to more effectively advance the health interests of future victims. To advance each of these interests, innovation and experimentation that is not carried out in a way that prepares the ground for more formal research does not constitute truly abductive work. Informal experimentation without rigorous data collection should be discouraged because it exposes individuals to interventions that have not been validated without facilitating the ability to determine the relative merits of those interventions (London, 2006*b*).

Second, part A of the first operational criterion requires that abductive work be carried out in human populations only when there are no other feasible means of learning about the relevant variables. If other means to generate the relevant information are feasible, these means should be preferred.

Finally, abductive work is by nature a process of forming possible causal models or theories from observations in particular cases. The value of those observations for informing those models is thus closely tied to their relevance to the condition that is being modeled. To serve their proper epistemic purpose, therefore, abductive activities should conform to the requirement set out in part B of the first operational criterion. For those aspects of abductive work that are motivated by a therapeutic, diagnostic, or prophylactic aspiration, this requirement should be fairly easy to enforce. In other cases, there must be either uncertainty or conflict in the expert community about whether the recipients of the novel intervention would be better off, with respect to their basic interests, receiving either a different intervention or no intervention at all.

The ability to apply this framework in practice will undoubtedly be enhanced by having a clear account of how to distinguish what I am calling basic interests from nonbasic interests (London, 2003, 2007*b*). Even without such clarification, however, this framework still provides substantive guidance to decision-makers. In particular, if uncertainty exists regarding how to classify the interest in question, the appropriate default requirement for research in this context is to treat it as basic and to apply the practical test.

An objection at this point might be that the integrative approach is not sufficiently responsive to the kind of exigencies that arise in the context of a severe public health emergency. For example, if the state has the power to quarantine some citizens in order to prevent the spread of infectious disease, the imperative to protect larger numbers of people from deadly or debilitating disease can justify the curtailment of the basic rights and liberties of some. Similarly, the effort to find effective interventions against novel contagions may require the knowing sacrifice of the basic interests of some in order to find the means to save more community members in the future.

In fact, nothing in the integrative approach would inhibit sound research from moving forward in an expeditious manner or prohibit the use of the most rigorous trial designs. This approach provides a strong justification for carrying out socially valuable research in all phases of public health emergency planning and response because the failure to carry out broad-based research activities in the face of substantial uncertainty or conflict can have important adverse consequences. In particular, the failure to gather data in a careful and systematic fashion makes it difficult to form a clear assessment of various methods of responding to a public health emergency. Providing unproved interventions to disaster victims can create a false sense of security on the part of both practitioners and recipients, and recognizing that different groups or entities are recommending different and potentially inconsistent responses to a problem can create the impression that public agencies do not know what they are doing or that they are purposefully deceiving at least a portion of the community. Moreover, if it is not clear to the community that research is being conducted in a way that is consistent with the principle of equality, community members may shun research participation and seek direct access to unproved interventions, thus creating the social perception that those who participate in research face a higher degree of risk than is actually the case or that the interests of some are being sacrificed, knowingly, for social gain.

Something like this might have occurred in the wake of the 2001 anthrax attacks. On December 21, 2001, the US Department of Health and Human Services published a list of three preventive treatment options for persons at risk for inhalational anthrax, some of whom had already completed the recommended 60-day regimen of antibiotics. These were (1) 60 days of antimicrobial prophylaxis, accompanied by monitoring for illness; (2) 100 days of antimicrobial prophylaxis, accompanied by monitoring for illness or adverse reactions; and (3) 100 days of antimicrobial prophylaxis plus three doses of anthrax vaccine administered over a 4-week period. The recommendation stated, "As an investigational new drug, the vaccine would need to be administered with the full informed consent of the individual as to possible risks. Individuals would also be asked to take part in a follow-up study measuring the effect of the vaccine when administered after exposure" (US Department of Health and Human Services, 2001).

Uncertainty about the relative merits of these options created the rationale for an important prospective trial (Doolan et al., 2007). Yet a failure to communicate the nature of this uncertainty and the importance of research to its resolution, along with differing perceptions about whether participation in the follow-up research was mandatory or optional, contributed to a perception of differential treatment between the predominantly white population of the Senate office building and the predominantly African American population of US postal workers. This perception of differential treatment at least raised the potential that those who were offered the investigational vaccine and who did not participate in the research follow-up may have perceived their "care" to involve a lower risk, whereas those who participated in the research may have perceived the research as having a higher risk. In actuality, if there was a difference, the opposite may have been the case.

Whether a particular trial design is justified in any instance will hinge on the nature of the uncertainty or conflict within the public health community and whether the practical test for the operational criterion is satisfied. However, the integrative approach would not permit knowingly withholding what is believed to be effective protections or interventions from research participants if doing so would have a detrimental impact on their basic interests. In this regard, it is less permissive than some forms of utilitarianism might be.

Any propensity to regard such permissiveness as a virtue should be tempered by a recognition of the following three points. First, creativity and ingenuity can often lead to studies that are of sufficient value as to alleviate the need to conduct trials in which such sacrifices are exacted from participants. Second, the history of research with human subjects is rife with claims that even ordinary burdens of sickness and disease are sufficient to justify sacrificing some at the altar of the greater good. This suggests that researchers have been too quick to make such claims in the past, and there is no reason to think that fear and trauma will make them more, rather than less, cautious and careful. Finally, in times of crisis, fear itself may impair the ability to estimate the true marginal value of the gains in time and possible lives saved from such efforts, given what we stand to lose in repudiating values of equal concern and respect that are essential to preserving trust in the research and public health system.

Not all public health research is designed to determine the best methods or interventions for public health emergency response. In some cases, researchers simply want to study phenomena that emerge primarily, or only, in the context of a public health crisis. To satisfy the first operational criterion, research activities that do not directly provide a method or intervention of crisis response to affected populations must not conflict with or impede the effective provision of such methods or interventions.

It is difficult to provide operationally precise guidance about the cumulative level of risk to which it is acceptable to allow participants to be exposed in such research. There is consensus that research risks should be "reasonable" in light of the value of the information the research is designed to generate (Emanuel et al., 2000; US Department of Health and Human Services, 2005). However, little operational guidance exists regarding how to determine the value of such information or how to trade it off against potential harms to research participants (Kaebnick, 2003). This is not a unique problem for the integrative approach; it is an open problem for research ethics in general (London, 2006*a*).

The second operational criterion for preserving equality represents a proposal for making such judgments in a more systematic and transparent manner. To generate a practical test for this criterion, stakeholders would have to identify comparison classes of activities in which individuals accept some incremental risks to their basic interests in order to benefit others or to advance the common good. Similarly, the risks associated with such activities should be viewed as necessary evils and not as desirable in their own right, as is often the case with dangerous pursuits such as rock climbing or motorcycle riding. To the extent possible, such activities should also be the subject of social oversight or review so that there is some reason to view their associated risks as socially acceptable.

I have proposed using the activities of public service professions, such as paramedics or firefighters, as possible reference classes (London, 2006*a*, 2007*b*). Other public service professions, such as social workers and even public health officials, could possibly be considered as well. The goal is to construct comparison classes that can be used to assure stakeholders that the incremental risks to the basic interests of participants that are associated with the purely research-related elements of a research initiative are no greater than, for instance, the incremental risks to the basic interests of social workers or paramedics encountered by members of those professions on a routine basis.

A public health emergency, however, is a special situation in which the basic interests of a population are at risk or have already been compromised. Moreover, as the experience with Hurricanes Katrina, Rita, and Sandy powerfully illustrated, public health crises can exacerbate preexisting social inequalities, exacting the harshest toll on marginalized, poor, or otherwise vulnerable groups. Special care must be taken, therefore, not to place significant additional burdens on the basic interests of disaster victims. Additionally, special care must be taken to ensure that the burdens of such research are not disproportionately borne by persons who are already socially, economically, or politically disadvantaged and that special protections are in place to ensure that the risks to individuals from such groups are minimized.

In light of these facts, it is best to err on the side of caution. Research on phenomena that emerge primarily in the context of a public health crisis should be evaluated with a risk-relative sliding scale, according to which the standard for justifying a level of incremental risk that rises above the minimal threshold is raised or lowered inversely with the severity of the public health crisis and the importance of the information that might be generated from the research.

On this proposal, there should exist a strong but defensible requirement that such research not subject participants to a cumulative, incremental level of risk that is more than minimal, where this is defined as "the probability and magnitude of harm or discomfort anticipated in the research are not greater in and of themselves than those ordinarily encountered in daily life or during the performance of routine physical or psychological examinations or tests" (US Department of Health and Human Services, 2005). To be clear, the appropriate comparison here should be to "daily life" and "routine physical or psychological examinations or tests" in the context of nonemergency situations and not to the level of risk that participants experience in the context of life during a public health emergency.

If a compelling case can be made that the research is necessary to generate information that will play an important role in shaping future emergency response activities, or in shaping research that will play such a role, then the threshold on acceptable risk might be raised to those that are routinely encountered by members of an appropriate service profession. In truly exceptional situations, such as research that would play a crucial role in addressing a deadly pandemic, it may be possible to raise the level of permissible risk to those that are encountered by first responders in the context of emergency response situations. Such steps should be taken with great caution and should be accompanied by strict oversight, a robust process of informed consent, and, to the greatest extent possible, extensive community consultation.

For such a recommendation to serve its social purpose in both protecting the interests of disaster victims and regulating socially consequential research, special care will have to be given to setting the relevant standards in a way that has clear, operational content (London, 2006*b*). It is also important that these standards be set in a way that reflects broad-based community input. Ideally, therefore, the content of the practical test for the second operational criterion should be determined during the planning and preparation phase of public health crisis response.

Making the Integrative Approach Operational: Conflicts in Resource Allocation

Conflicts in resource allocation can occur at various stages of emergency planning and response and at a variety of levels. In addition, the responsibility for avoiding or mitigating them often falls on a diverse range of stakeholders. Some of the most profound conflicts in resource allocation occur at the level of priority setting. With public health research being a resource-intensive activity, a general question arises about how much of a society's scarce social resources should be allocated to funding research. Once this question is addressed, research priorities must then be set so that scarce social resources can be directed at the most important research questions.

It should be emphasized that some of the most crucial conflicts in resource allocation represent problems that fall outside of research ethics and within the scope of a general theory of distributive justice. As such, they fall outside the scope of this chapter. Because it does not provide a framework for addressing larger issues of distributive justice, the integrative approach can only provide guidance about how to address a much narrower and more local set of conflicts in resource allocation.

For example, within this framework, it is clear that even if research focuses on generating new interventions, policies, or plans for public health emergency response, it can in some cases undermine the capacity of public health institutions to serve their proper social function. This is most likely to occur when such research activities (1) focus on crisis events that have a low probability of occurring and (2) are directed at studying interventions, policies, or procedures that do not enhance the capacity of the public health infrastructure more generally or do not enhance its capacity to deal with a broad range of more common emergency situations.

In the most extreme cases, poor planning at the level of priority setting can create research programs that are self-defeating. For example, a successful attack on a major US city using a weaponized strain of smallpox could potentially have devastating consequences for vast numbers of Americans. A research program that investigates vaccines or other treatments whose applicability is limited to such weaponized forms of smallpox would be self-defeating if it diverts scarce public health resources from the existing public health infrastructure, thereby degrading its capacity to apply in practice any knowledge that might be gained from such focused research programs. The problem here is not simply the low probability of such an attack, because it may be reasonable to take steps to prevent or mitigate the impact of even low-probability events if their consequences would be sufficiently grave. Rather, the point is that the effective application of new knowledge, strategies, and interventions requires a public health infrastructure with the capacity to implement them effectively on a widespread basis. A robust public health infrastructure is also essential to detecting, containing, and addressing an array of threats to the health of communities that arise on a more regular basis.

Effective preservation of the public's health depends on the dynamic interaction between the health needs of the community; the social, political, and natural environment; and the institutions, policies, and programs that are designed to meet those needs under a broad range of conditions. For this reason, the integrative approach directs stakeholders to set research priorities in a way that enhances the capacity of the public health infrastructure to deal with a wide spectrum of public health threats. Research programs that have a synergistic effect on the capacity of public health institutions to meet a variety of challenges to the public's health should be given priority over research programs that seek to provide interventions that are narrowly targeted to address low-probability events.

Conflicts in resource allocation can occur at more local levels as well. For instance, when deployed in response to a particular public health emergency, personnel from an agency such as the CDC may identify a unique research opportunity. Even when such research can be justified on the account described here, such fortuitous research opportunities can pose conflicts in resource allocation to the extent that they divert time, energy, and other resources away from the primary mission of public health crisis response.

It is particularly salient in the integrative approach that institutions such as the CDC play a special role in the social division of labor as it relates to public health emergency response. Special powers and prerogatives are granted to such agencies so they can more effectively preserve the basic health interests of community members. Although it is important to pursue research opportunities, this must be done in a way that does not compromise the fundamental goals of emergency response. As such, the personnel of such agencies should pursue fortuitous research opportunities only if they can do so without compromising the goal of safeguarding the basic health interests of the affected population.

In some cases, these goals can be reconciled by expanding the pie: researchers can work additional hours, or additional resources can be allocated to the fortuitous research activity. Where the pie cannot be so expanded, however, it may not be permissible for personnel from agencies with a special role in public health emergency response to pursue the research opportunity. This does not mean, however, that it would be impermissible for agents who do not have such special obligations to pursue the research in question.

It may thus be appropriate to create an institutional mechanism through which such fortuitous opportunities could be publicized to a broader community of researchers. For instance, research funds could be set aside for such opportunities. A granting mechanism could be designated that would create a registry of researchers organized by research topic and geographic location. When a fortuitous research opportunity emerges, the registry could be searched for researchers with an established record of research in the relevant area who might be in sufficient proximity to respond in a timely manner. Researchers could then submit a research protocol to the granting agency for special review.

However, this particular proposal would only apply to cases in which the public health emergency in question is of a scale and a magnitude that it can be effectively addressed by the activities of the social agencies that are charged with responding to such crises or in which the crisis is such that the provision of crisis response must be left to personnel with appropriate training or protective equipment. If a public health emergency rises to the level of a humanitarian crisis, persons who are capable of doing so may have an overriding duty to contribute to crisis relief. Such a duty may simply trump the imperative to carry out fortuitous research, no matter who seeks to conduct it.

The merits of any such proposal would hinge crucially on how such practical details are worked out in actual practice, but the motivation for this general proposal is drawn from the central tenets of the integrative approach: namely, to create an institutional framework within which labor can be divided among identifiable parties so that important public health research can be conducted in a way that does not compromise the goals of effective public health emergency response.

References

Anderson, E. S. (1999). What is the point of equality? *Ethics*, *109*, 287–337.

Blanchard, J. C., Haywood, Y., Stein, B. D., Tanielian, T. L., Stoto, M., & Lurie, N. (2005). In their own words: Lessons learned from those exposed to anthrax. *American Journal of Public Health*, *95*, 489–495.

Centers for Disease Control and Prevention (CDC). (1999). *Guidelines for defining public health research and public health non-research.* Revised October 4, 1999. Available at http://www.cdc.gov/od/science/integrity/docs/defining-public-health-research-non-research-1999.pdf.

Centers for Disease Control and Prevention (CDC). (2010). *Distinguishing public health research and public health nonresearch*. Available at http://www.cdc.gov/od/science/integrity/docs/cdc-policy-distinguishing-public-health-research-nonresearch.pdf.

Council for International Organizations of Medical Sciences. (2002). *International ethical guidelines for biomedical research involving human subjects*. Geneva: World Health Organization Press.

Doolan, D. L., Freilich, D. A., Brice, G. T., Burgess, T. H., Berzins, M. P., Bull, R. L., . . . Martin, G. J. (2007). The US Capitol bioterrorism anthrax exposures: Clinical epidemiological and immunological characteristics. *Journal of Infectious Diseases, 195*, 174–184.

Emanuel, E. J., Wendler, D., & Grady, C. (2000). What makes clinical research ethical? *Journal of the American Medical Association, 283*, 2701–2710.

Evans, E. L., & London, A. J. (2006). Equipoise and the criteria for reasonable action. *Journal of Law, Medicine & Ethics, 34*, 441–450.

Freedman, B. (1987). Equipoise and the ethics of clinical research. *New England Journal of Medicine, 317*, 141–145.

Freedman, B. (1990). Placebo controlled trials and the logic of clinical purpose. *IRB. Review of Human Subjects Research, 12*, 1–6.

Freimuth, V. S., Quinn, S. C., Thomas, S. B., Cole, G., Zook, E., & Duncan T. (2001). African Americans' views on research and the Tuskegee syphilis study. *Social Science & Medicine, 52*, 797–808.

Fried, C. (1974). *Medical experimentation: Personal integrity and social policy*. Amsterdam: North-Holland.

Gifford, F. (1986). The conflict between randomized clinical trials and the therapeutic obligation. *Journal of Medicine and Philosophy, 11*, 347–366.

Gifford, F. (1995). Community-equipoise and the ethics of randomized clinical trials. *Bioethics, 9*, 127–184.

Gifford, F. (2000). Freedman's "clinical equipoise" and "sliding-scale all-dimensions-considered equipoise." *Journal of Medicine and Philosophy, 25*, 399–426.

Hellman, D. (2002). Evidence, belief, and action: The failure of equipoise to resolve the ethical tension in the randomized clinical trial. *Journal of Law, Medicine & Ethics, 30*, 375–380.

Kadane, J. B. (Ed.). (1996). *Bayesian methods and ethics in a clinical trial design*. New York: Wiley.

Kaebnick, G. E. (2003). From the Editor: No wonder research ethics is confusing. *Hastings Center Report, 33*, 2.

Levi, I. (1986). *Hard choices: Decision making under unresolved conflict.* New York: Cambridge University Press.
London, A. J. (2003). Threats to the common good: Biochemical weapons and human subjects' research. *Hastings Center Report, 33*, 17–25.
London, A. J. (2005). Justice and the human development approach to international research. *Hastings Center Report, 35*, 24–37.
London, A. J. (2006a). Reasonable risks in clinical research: A critique and a proposal for the integrative approach. *Statistics in Medicine, 25*, 2869–2885.
London, A. J. (2006b). Cutting surgical practice at the joints: Individuating and assessing surgical procedures. In A. M. Rietsma & J. D. Moreno (Eds.), *Ethical guidelines for innovative surgery* (pp. 19–52). Hagerstown, MD: University Publishing Group.
London, A. J. (2007a). Clinical equipoise: Foundational requirement or fundamental error. In B. Steinbock (Ed.), *Oxford handbook of bioethics* (pp. 571–596). New York: Oxford University Press.
London, A. J. (2007b). Two dogmas of research ethics and the integrative approach to human-subjects research. *Journal of Medicine and Philosophy, 32*, 99–116.
MacQueen, K. M., & Huehler, J. W. (2004). Ethics, practice, and research in public health. *American Journal of Public Health, 96*, 928–931.
Marquis, D. (1983). Leaving therapy to chance. *Hastings Center Report, 13*, 40–47.
McCallum, J. M., Arekere, D. M., Green, B. L., Katz, R. V., & Rivers, B. M. (2006). Awareness and knowledge of the U.S. Public Health Service syphilis study at Tuskegee: Implications for biomedical research. *Journal of Health Care for the Poor and Underserved, 17*, 716–733.
Miller, F. G., & Brody, H. (2003). A critique of clinical equipoise: Therapeutic misconception in the ethics of clinical trials. *Hastings Center Report, 33*, 19–28.
Miller F. G., & Brody, H. (2007). Clinical equipoise and the incoherence of research ethics. *Journal of Medicine and Philosophy, 32*, 151–165.
Miller, P. B., & Weijer, C. (2003). Rehabilitating equipoise. *Kennedy Institute of Ethics Journal, 13*, 93–118.
Muller, M. P., McGeer, A., Straus, S. E., Hawryluck, L., & Gold, W. L. (2004). Clinical trials and novel pathogens: Lessons learned from SARS. *Emerging Infectious Diseases, 10*, 389–394.

Nussbaum, M. (2000). *Women and human development: The capabilities approach*. New York: Cambridge University Press.

Quinn, S., Thomas, T., & McAllister, C. (2005). Postal workers' perspectives on communication during the anthrax attack. *Biosecurity and Bioterrorism, 3*, 207–215.

Rawls, J. (1971). *A theory of justice*. Cambridge, MA: Harvard University Press.

Rawls, J. (1982). Social unity and the primary goods. In A. Sen & B. Williams (Eds.), *Utilitarianism and beyond* (pp. 159–185). New York: Cambridge University Press.

Sen, A. (1982). Equality of what? In A. Sen (Ed.), *Choice, welfare, and measurement* (pp. 353–369). Cambridge, MA: Harvard University Press.

Stockman, L. J., Bellamy, R., & Garner, P. (2006). SARS: Systematic review of treatment effects. *PLoS Medicine, 3*, e343.

US Department of Health and Human Services. (2001). Statement by the Department of Health And Human Services regarding additional options for preventive treatment for those exposed to inhalational anthrax (Press release). Washington DC: US Department of Health and Human Services. Available at http://archive.hhs.gov/news/press/2001pres/20011218.html.

US Department of Health and Human Services. (2005). Protection of Human Subjects. *45*, CFR §46.102(d).

Working Group on "Governance Dilemmas" in Bioterrorism Response. (2004). Leading during bioattacks and epidemics with the public's trust and help. *Biosecurity and Bioterrorism, 2*, 25–40.

Index

Page numbers followed by *t* and *b* indicate tables and boxes, respectively. Numbers followed by n indicate notes.

abductive phase of inquiry, 248–249
abductive research, 246–249
abuse: prevention of, 40
accountability, 65
  conditions that ensure, 128–129
  to public, 167–168
  for reasonableness, 127–132, 166
advance planning, 38–39, 46–47
African Americans, 23–24, 50, 52–53, 232
aggregate health: maximization of, 115
AIDS, 68, 74, 75
all-hazards approach, xxi
American Medical Association (AMA), 67–68
American Public Health Association, xvii
anthrax attacks, xix, 107, 232, 250–251
Antiterrorism and Effective Death Penalty Act of 1996 (P.L. 104–132, Section 511), xix
antiviral drugs, 121–123
appeals processes, 34–35
Aristotle, 230
Arras, John, ix, x, xxvii
Asian Americans, 52–53
ASPR. *see* Office of the Assistant Secretary for Preparedness and Response (DHHS)
assessment
  cultural, 51
  ethical, 90n13
assistance
  public assistance programs, 143
  recovery, 40
assistance delayed, 40
at-risk persons, 50
audit, community, 51
authoritarianism
  benevolent, 59, 65
  emergency exception for, 65
autism: people with, 46

basic health interests, 222–223
basic interests, 237–238
Beasts of the Southern Wild, 44
beneficence, 192, 212n5, 214n12
benefit promotion, 13
benevolent authoritarianism, 59, 65
best outcomes, 113
biodefense, 107
bioterrorism, xix, 11
Bioterrorism Preparedness and Response Program (CDC), xix
blogs, 161
budget restrictions, 132

Camus, Albert, 77
Canada, 74
caretakers, 55
case study, 162–164, 180–181
Centers for Disease Control and Prevention (CDC), ix, 18
  Advisory Committee to the Director (ACD), ix, xxvi, xxvii
  Bioterrorism Preparedness and Response Program, xix
  Ethics Subcommittee of the Advisory Committee to the Director, ix, xxvii
  public health ethics, xxvi–xxvii
  Public Health Ethics Committee (PHEC), xxvi–xxvii, xxxiin2
  roles and responsibilities, xxv–xxvi, 257
Chernobyl, Russia, 75
child care workers, 55
children, 147
China, 66–67, 72
citizenship, responsible, 14
citizens' panels or juries, 170, 171–172
civic commitment, 14
civic obligations, 77–82, 186–219
civic participation, 59–61, 78–80
civic partnership, 37–38
civic practice, 2, 9–14, 41–42, 59–61, 71, 72, 186–219
  compass points for, 12–14
  fostering, 78–80
civic renewal, 11
civil liberties, 17–22
climate change, xx
code of ethics, xvii
cognitive disabilities: persons with, 142, 144–146
collaborative partnerships, 178–179
Common Rule, 230
communication
  about emergency planning, 57–58
  in emergency preparedness, 56–66
  with public, 158–159, 161–162
  recommendations for preparedness planning for vulnerable populations, 53
  during response, 61–62
  spectrum of, 57–59
  transparent, 57–59, 62
communitarianism, 24
community, 175–176
community activists, 61

community assets, 51
community consent, 176
community consultations, 58
community groups, 177
community health, 176
community obligations, 191, 194–195
community organization, 79–80
community participation, 13–14, 80, 161–162
community partners, 50
community prioritization policy, 158
community relations, 158–159, 177–178, 181
community representatives, 60–61
community resilience and empowerment, 13–14
community trust, 178–179
compass points, 12–14
compliance
  with public health authority, 65
  voluntary versus mandatory, 20–22
conflict(s), 245
  in goals, 239–255
  of obligations, 202–203
  in resource allocation, 255–258
consensus conferences, 171
consequentialism, 110, 113–114, 210n2
consultation, 156
  community, 58
  for public engagement, 161–162
consumerism, 9–12, 77–78
contractual obligations, 193, 210n2, 216n24
cooptation, 60–61
coronavirus, 245
cultural appropriate information, 52
cultural appropriate interventions, 47–48
cultural assessment, 51
cultural differences, 52–53, 132

DALYs. *see* disability-adjusted life years
Daniels, Norman, 166
Dark Winter exercise, xix
databases, special-needs, 49, 50
decision-making, 159
  effects of, 84–85
  ethical considerations, 84–85
  fair, deliberative process of, 127–132
  publicity in, 33–34
  transparency in, 33–34
Defense Against Weapons of Mass Destruction Act (P.L. 104–201) (Nunn-Lugar-Domenici Act), xix, xxv
deliberations, 24–25, 127–132, 156, 168–170
  benefits of, 168–169
  about justice, 24–27
  normative conditions for, 170
  primary considerations for, 170
  proliferation of procedures, 169
  public, 157–158, 170, 182
  types or methods of, 170
democratic participation, 36

Department of Health and Human Services (DHHS), xix
  Office of the Assistant Secretary for Preparedness and Response (ASPR), xxvi
  recommended preventive treatment options for anthrax, 250–251
  roles and responsibilities of, xxvi
disabilities: persons with
  recommendations for preparedness planning for, 52–53
  vulnerability to losses, 147
disability-adjusted life years (DALYs), 29, 105, 113
disaster planning, 25
dissemination, 156
distributive fairness, 132–133
distributive justice, 13, 118
division of labor, 114, 257
drugs, antiviral, xix, 121–123
due diligence, 85–86
duty-based theories of justice, 30–31
duty of personal care, 227–228
duty to care, 199–206, 209, 212n5, 215n20
duty to treat, 215n20
"Duty to Treat or Right to Refuse" (Daniels), 199–200

earthquakes, xx
economically vulnerable populations, 141–144
  risk of loss, 138–139
  vulnerability to losses, 147
efficiency, 27–28, 28–31
egalitarianism, 24
emergency communications, 56–66
emergency exceptions, 9–12, 65–66
emergency excuse, 65
emergency interventions
  availability of, 83
  bases for, 83
  effects on ethical values, 83–84
  goals of, 82–83
  ladder of, 18–19, 90n12
emergency preparedness and response, 9–12
  case study, 162–164, 180–181
  as civic practice, 10–14, 41–42, 59–61, 72, 186–219
  communication in, 56–66
  compass points for, 12–14
  as continuum, 106–108
  evaluation of, 85
  goals of, 221–227
  implementation of, 85–86
  maximization in, 110–115
  versus other health needs, 106–110
  participation in, 56–66
  personal obligations in, 186–219
  phases of, 38–40
  as political undertaking, 164–172
  professional obligations in, 66–77, 186–219
  public engagement in, 155–185
  public health, xxi, xxii–xxv
  questions to ask, 84

recommendations for, 82–86
research in, 220–261
resource allocation for, 104–134
success of, 225
volunteers during, 62–65
vulnerable populations, 135–154
emergency transportation, 54–55
shelters, 54–55
empirical evidence, 206–207
empowerment, 13–14, 80
enforcement, 129
environmental hazards, 141
equality
moral equal protection, 148, 150–151
preserving, 239–241, 240*b*, 243*b*, 252–253
principle of, 238–239, 238*b*
equal liberty, 13
equipoise, 227–228
equity, 105–106
justice as, 27–28, 31–33
versus maximization, 115–126
Escherichia coli contamination, xix–xx, 11
Ethical Guidance for Public Health Emergency Preparedness and Response: Highlighting Ethics and Values in a Vital Public Health Service, xxvii
Ethical Guidelines in Pandemic Influenza (Kinlaw, Barrett, & Levine), xxvii
ethics
assessment, 90n13
considerations for, 84–85, 90n13
ethics, 1–103
goals, 41–42
importance of, 4–12
organizational, 174–175
perspectives, 155–185
professional, 174
public health, xvii, xxvi–xxvii
questions to ask, 84
recommendations for emergency planning, 82–86
values, 83–84
Ethics Subcommittee of the Advisory Committee to the Director (CDC), ix
ethnic minorities
recommendations for preparedness planning for, 50
special needs of, 45
evacuations, 54, 89n9
evaluation, 85
evidence
empirical, 206–207
responding to, 206–209
exceptionalism, 106–108

fair chances, 113
fair-minded parties, 129
fairness, 114, 127–128, 182
accountability for reasonableness, 127–132
for all, 31–33
distributive, 132–133
need for, 127–132
requirements for fair processes, 33–36
Federal Emergency Management Agency (FEMA), xix

federalism, 118
Federal Response Plan, xxv
FEMA. *see* Federal Emergency Management Agency
fiduciary duty, 227–228
financially vulnerable populations, 141–144
  risk of loss, 138–139
  vulnerability to losses, 147
firefighters, 63, 141, 253
food supply, xix–xx
forums or town hall meetings, 170–172
France, 89n8
fraud, 40
Freedman, Benjamin, 227
Fried, Charles, 227
The Future of the Public Health in the 21st Century (IOM), 173

geographically isolated persons, 48, 141
geographically vulnerable populations, 141
"God" committee, 122–123

H1N1 infections, xxv, 126
H5N1 infections, 109–110
Haiti, xx
harm prevention, 14–17
harm reduction, 13, 16
hazard mitigation, 80
health, aggregate, 115
health care providers, 141, 186
health care workers, 141
  moral obligations of, 73
  obligations of, 66–77
  in SARS epidemic, 76
  scenarios, 186, 187
  victims of SARS, 74
health interests, basic, 222–223
health literacy, 80
health measures, 112–114
health ministries, 50
health needs, 106–110
health professionals. *see also* public health professionals (PHPs)
  obligations of, 66–77, 186–219
  in SARS epidemic, 76
heroism, 213n6
Hippocratic Oath, 174
Hispanics, 52–53
HIV/AIDS, 75, 168
hoarding, 125–126
Homeland Security Act of 2002 (P. L. 107–296), xxv
Homeland Security Policy Directive-5, xxv
Homeland Security Presidential Directive (HSP)-21, xxv
Hong Kong, 74
human rights, 13
human subjects research, 223, 251–252
Hurricane Katrina, xx, xxv, 15, 23–24, 43, 44, 54, 74, 138–139, 253
Hurricane Rita, 253

inclusiveness, 13, 56–57, 59–61, 65–66
individualism, 7–8, 17–22, 182
infectious disease, 55
influenza
  case study, 162–164, 180–181

Ethical Guidelines in Pandemic Influenza (Kinlaw, Barrett, & Levine), xxvii
pandemic, 11, 26–27, 68
information exchange, 177, 181
informed consent, 46
infrastructure, xxi
Institute of Medicine (IOM), xviii, 1, 173, 174–175
integrative approach, xxxi, 220–261
criteria for preserving equality, 239–241, 240*b*, 243*b*, 252–253
as operational, 239–255, 255–258
to research, 234–258
intellectual disabilities: persons with, 46, 144–146
International Federation of Red Cross and Red Crescent Societies, 147
interpreters, 52
intuition, 6
isolated persons, 47

Japan, xx
Jennings, Bruce, ix, xxvii
Johns Hopkins University, 18
judgment, 5–6
juries, 171–172
justice, 38–40, 104–134
alternative approaches to, 30–31
deliberating about, 24–27
distributive, 13, 118
duty-based theories of, 30–31
as efficiency, 27–31
as equity, 27–28, 31–33
non-consequentialist theories of, 30–31
during planning, 38–39
prioritarian, 147–149
during recovery, 39–40
during resource allocation, 22–40
justification, public, 164–172

Kant, Immanuel, 212–213n5
King, Martin Luther, 36

labor: division of, 114, 257
ladder of intervention, 18–19, 90n12
language issues, 52
lawsuits: fear of, 63–64
leadership, 178
learning communities, 87n2
learning organizations, 87n2
least restrictive alternatives, 18–19
legislation. *see specific acts, laws*
legitimacy, 169
conditions for, 65
political, 169
of public health officials, 65
through stakeholder involvement, 130–131
legitimacy problem, 127–128
libertarianism, 24
liberty
equal, 13
individual, 17–22
life saving, 14–17, 113
linguistically appropriate information, 52
local knowledge, 48, 53
local services, 214n16, 256–257

loss
  cascading, 142–144
  risk of, 137–139
  types of, 136–137

Maginot Line, 89n8
mandatory compliance, 20–22
mapping community assets, 51
marginalized populations, 84
marketing, 158–159, 181
martyrdom, 75
mass media, 161
maximization, 105–106, 110–115
  of aggregate health, 115
  arguments for, 114
  versus equity, 115–126
  of life years vs lives saved, 113
  of QALYs vs DALYs, 113
MDR-TB. *see* multidrug-resistant tuberculosis
measures of health, 112–114
medical care, 63
medically vulnerable populations, 138, 140, 141
medical resources
  allocation of, 158
  stockpiling, xix, 119, 125–126
medications, 121–123
medics, 63
mental illness: persons with, 45, 141
mild cognitive disabilities: persons with, 46
minorities, 147
Model State Emergency Health Powers Act, 18, 64, 89n11
moral equal protection, 148, 150–151
moral obligations, 67, 73, 189, 192–193, 196–199, 205–206, 210n1, 211n4
multidrug-resistant tuberculosis (MDR-TB), xix–xx

National Incident Management System (NIMS), xxvi
National Response Framework (NRF), xxv–xxvi
national stockpile of pharmaceuticals and vaccines, xix, 126
natural disasters, 106–107
natural vulnerability, 140
necessity, 18
New Orleans, LA, 44
NIMS. *see* National Incident Management System
9/11 (September 11, 2001 terrorist attacks), xix, 15, 63, 81–82
non-consequentialist theories of justice, 30–31
nonmaleficence, 192, 212n5, 214n12
norms and values, 3
NRF. *see* National Response Framework
Nuffield Council on Bioethics, 90n12, 175–176
Nunn-Lugar-Domenici Act. *see* Defense Against Weapons of Mass Destruction Act (P.L. 104- 201)
nurses. *see* health care workers

objective obligations, 197
obligations, 118
  civic, 77–82, 186–219
  community, 191, 194–195
  concept of, 188–191, 196–199, 210n2
  conflicts of, 202–203
  contractual, 193, 210n2, 216n24
  fulfilling, 206–209
  general, 192
  moral, 67, 73, 189, 192–193, 196–199, 205–206, 210n1, 211n4
  natural, 192
  nonconsensual, 193
  objective, 197
  parent-child, 197
  personal, 186–219
  prima facie, 188, 191, 200, 202, 203, 209
  professional, xxiv, 66–77, 186–219
  pro tanto, 211n3
  of reciprocity, 214n8
  role, 193, 194, 209
  to self, 214n11
  societal, 72, 73
  special, 192
  subjective, 197
  therapeutic, 227–228
  types of, 189, 192–196, 211–213n5
Office of the Assistant Secretary for Preparedness and Response (ASPR) (DHHS), xxvi
Oklahoma City, Oklahoma attacks, xviii–xix
opportunity costs, 88n5
organizational ethics, 174–175
oseltamivir, 109–110, 126
overgeneralization, 52–53

Pandemic and All-Hazards Preparedness (PAHPA) Act of 2006 (P. L. 109–417), xxv
pandemic influenza, xxvii, 11, 26–27, 68
paramedics, 253
parent-child obligations, 197
partnerships, collaborative, 178–179
paternalism, 6–7, 59, 60–61, 65
personal obligations, 186–219
personal responsibility, 77–82
pharmaceuticals, xix, 121–123
philosophy, public, 166
Photovoice, 161
PHPs. *see* public health professionals
physical disabilities: persons with, 46, 52–53, 141
physicians, 141, 186
  plague doctors, 76–77
  scenarios, 186
place-based research, 16, 87n2
plague doctors, 76–77
planning, 108–110
  advance planning, 38–39
  all-hazards approach to, xxi
  disaster planning, 25
  justice issues in, 38–39
  for meeting special needs of vulnerable populations, 42
  for problems, 206–209
  recommendations for, 49–56
  for vulnerable populations, 49–56

planning and preparedness phase, 222
planning cells, 171
planning phase, 7–8, 12, 20, 38–39, 42, 47, 66
pluralism, 168–169
police, 63, 141
political legitimacy, 169
political responsibility, 182
political undertakings, 164–172
poor. *see* financially vulnerable populations
postal workers, 232
post-crisis transition phase, 223
preparedness, xxi, 87n3. *see also* public health emergency preparedness and response
preparedness planning. *see* planning
prima facie obligations, 191, 200, 202, 203, 209
Principles of the Ethical Practice of Public Health (Public Health Code of Ethics), xxx, 155, 164, 174–182
prioritarian justice, 147–149
prioritization, 14–15, 26–27, 120–123, 211–213n5
  community policy, 158
  giving priority to worst-off, 147–149
  during recovery, 39–40
private dilemmas, 80–82
private stockpiling, 125–126
professional duty, 76–77
professional ethics, 174
professionalism, 14, 214n8
professional obligations, xxiv, 66–77, 186–219
pro tanto obligations, 211n3
public assistance programs, 143
public consent, 175–176
public deliberations, 182. *see also* deliberations
  need for, 157–158
  types or methods of, 170
public education, 80
public engagement, 36, 58, 155–185
  case study, 162–164, 180–181
  deliberative, evidence-based approach to, 182
  goal of, 160
  as political undertaking, 164–172
  as social undertaking, 172–180
  techniques for, 161–162
public forums, 170–172
public goods, 116–118
public health
  basic health interests, 222–223
  climate change threats to, xx
  definition of, xviii, xx–xxi, 164
  public consent in, 175–176
  reemergence of, xviii–xxii
  role of, 151–152
public health agencies, 157, 174–175
public health and medical preparedness, xxii–xxiii
public health authority, 65
Public Health Code of Ethics *(Principles of the Ethical Practice of Public Health)*, xxx, 155, 164, 174–182

public health emergencies:
research during, 220–261, 240*b*, 243*b*, 244*b*
public health emergency preparedness and response, xxii–xxv. *see also* emergency preparedness and response
activities, xxiii
case study, 162–164, 180–181
civic obligations in, 186–219
consensus points, xxi
current frameworks for, 227–234
definition of, xxii
ethical aspects of, 1–103
ethical perspectives on, 155–185
personal obligations in, 186–219
professional obligations in, xxiv, 66–77, 186–219
public engagement in, 155–185
research in, 220–261
resource allocation for, 104–134
vulnerable populations, 135–154
public health ethics, xvii, xxvi–xxvii
Public Health Leadership Society, 174–175
public health measures, 55
public health officials, 157, 168, 173–174, 178, 181–182
legitimacy of, 65
as reference classes, 253
public health practices, 155–159
ethical perspectives in, 155–185
foundations for, 173–174
public health professionals (PHPs), 14, 198–199, 213–214nn7–8
duty of care in emergencies, 199–206, 209
ethics of, 174
obligations of, xxiv, 66–77, 186–219
public health research, 252
abductive, 246–249
criteria for preserving equality, 239–241, 240*b*, 243*b*, 252–253
during emergencies, 220–261
evaluation of, 227–234
human subjects research, 251–252
integrative approach to, 234–258
practical tests for, 243–244, 244*b*, 246
Public Health Security and Bioterrorism Preparedness and Response Act of 2002 (P. L. 107–188), xxv
public health services, 157–158
public hearings, 170, 171
publicity, 33–34, 128, 130, 170
public justification, 164–172
Public Law 104–132. *see* Antiterrorism and Effective Death Penalty Act of 1996
Public Law 104–201. *see* Defense Against Weapons of Mass Destruction Act (Nunn-Lugar-Domenici Act)
Public Law 107–188. *see* Public Health Security and Bioterrorism Preparedness and Response Act of 2002

Public Law 107–296. *see* Homeland Security Act of 2002
Public Law 109–417. *see* Pandemic and All-Hazards Preparedness (PAHPA) Act of 2006
public participation, 37–38, 53, 169
public philosophy, 166
public relations, 170, 172–180
public service professionals, 253
public transparency, 13
public transportation, 143
public trust, xxi, 172–180
Putnam, Robert, 90n13

quality-adjusted life years (QALYs), 29–30, 105, 113
quality control, 64
questions to ask, 84

racial minorities
- recommendations for preparedness planning for, 50
- special needs of, 45

rationing, 33–34, 122–123
Rawls, John, 235
reasonableness: accountability for, 127–132
reciprocity, 123, 214n8
recovery assistance, 40
recovery phase, 7–8, 12, 39–40, 42, 47
recovery workers, 141
reference classes, 253
refugees, 147
registries, 49
relevance, 34, 129, 130
rescue: rule of, 14–15
research
- abductive, 246–249
- criteria for preserving equality, 239–241, 240*b*, 243*b*, 252–253
- criteria for success, 225
- effects of, 223
- frameworks for evaluation of, 227–234
- human subjects research, 223, 251–252
- integrative approach to, 234–258
- place-based, 16, 87n2
- practical tests for, 243–244, 244*b*, 246
- during public health emergencies, 220–261
- Tuskegee syphilis study, 232

resilience, 87n3
- community, 13–14
- social, 88n3

resource allocation, 22–40, 104–134, 158, 226
- conflicts in, 255–258
- stockpiling, xix, 104–134

respect for individual interests, 17–22, 182
respiratory illness: case study, 162–164, 180–181
response phase, 12, 42, 46, 222. *see also* emergency preparedness and response
- communication during, 61–62
- justice issues in, 38–39
- mid-course corrections during, 90
- participation during, 62–65

responsibility, 117
  civic, 80
  fostering, 78–80
  personal, 77–82
  political, 182
  shared, 116–118
responsible citizenship, 14
restraints, 46
revisability, 129
ribairin, 245
rights, human, 13
risk communication, 58, 181
risk profiles, 137–139
role obligations, 193, 194, 209
rule of rescue, 14–15
rule utilitarianism, 234

Sandy (storm), 74
SARS. *see* severe acute respiratory syndrome
saving lives, 14–17, 113
scenarios, 186, 187
scientific literacy, 80
security, 87n3
separateness of persons, 231
September 11, 2001 terrorist attacks (9/11), xix, 15, 63, 81–82
severe acute respiratory syndrome (SARS), xix–xx, 68, 74
  in China, 66–67, 72, 76
  mortality rate, 74
  Taiwan outbreak, 207
  Toronto outbreak, 73, 206–207, 245
Shang-An, Taiwan, 79
shared responsibility, 116–118
simulation exercises, xix
social aspects, 156
social capital, 78
social distancing, 55
social division of labor, 257
social justice, 135
socially isolated persons, 48
socially vulnerable populations, 48, 140
social marketing, 158–159, 181
social media, 161
social networking, 161
social norms, 158–159
social psychology, 169
social resilience, 88n3
social trust, 233
social undertakings, 172–180
social utility, 231
social workers, 253
social worth, 109
societal obligations, 72, 73
socioeconomic vulnerability, 140
Spanish-speaking residents, 52
special needs: persons with
  identification of, 49, 54
  recommendations for preparedness planning for, 52–53
  vulnerable populations, 41–56
special-needs databases, 49, 50
stakeholders, 130–132
  definition of, 84
  identification of, 84
  involvement of, 36, 130–131
standards of care, 63–64
stereotyping, 52–53
stockpiling, xix, 104–134
  argument for, 115–126
  goals of, 119

stockpiling (*Cont.*)
national stockpile of pharmaceuticals and vaccines, xix, 126
objectives of, 119
for pandemics, 119
private, 125–126
street science, 6, 79–80
subjective obligations, 197
Superdome (New Orleans), 23–24
supererogation, 70, 213n6
surveillance and early warning systems, 79–80

Taiwan, China, 79–80, 207
terrorism, xviii–xix
9/11 (September 11, 2001 attacks), xix, 15, 63, 81–82
victims of, 141
therapeutic obligations, 227–228
time management, 85–86
Tokyo, Japan attacks, xviii–xix
TOPOFF1 exercise, xix
Toronto, Canada, 73, 206–207, 245
tort liability, 64
town hall meetings, 170–172
transition phase, post-crisis, 223
transparency, 56, 57–59, 65–66
in decision-making, 33–34
definition of, 89n10
provisions for, 56–57
public, 13, 167–168
rules of thumb for, 62
transportation
emergency, 54–55
public, 143
triage, 125
trust, 174
public, 172–180
social, 233
tsunamis, xx
tuberculosis, multidrug-resistant (MDR-TB), xix–xx
Tuskegee syphilis study, 232
Twitter, 161
uncertainty, 108–110, 244
utilitarianism, 24, 29, 110, 111, 231–234
vaccines, xix, 119–121, 126
values, 3, 83–84
ventilators, 124–125
Vietnam, 74
Vietnamese communities (Gulf Coast), 47
virtue perspective, 69–70
voluntarism, 192–194, 197
voluntary compliance, 20–22, 49
volunteers, 62–65
vulnerability
attributes of, 136–152
concept of, 42–45, 136–152
economic or financial, 141–144
elevated, 141–142, 147
forms of, 43–44
geographic, 48, 141
to loss, 136–137, 142–144
medical, 138, 140, 141
moral relevance of, 147
natural, 140
risk factors for, 142–143
socially situated, 140
types of loss, 136–137

variations in, 142–144
varieties of, 146–147

vulnerable populations, 135–154
  definition of, 147
  examples, 144–147
  identification of, 49, 54, 84
  recommendations for preparedness planning for, 49–56
  risk profiles, 137–139
  special needs of, 41–56

waste, fraud, and abuse, 40
welfarism, 110
West Nile virus, xix–xx
women, 147
Working Group on "Governance Dilemmas" in Bioterrorism Response, 233
World Health Organization (WHO), 109–110
World Trade Center attacks, xviii–xix, 15, 63, 81–82
worst-off groups, 115, 147–149

www.ingramcontent.com/pod-product-compliance
Ingram Content Group UK Ltd.
Pitfield, Milton Keynes, MK11 3LW, UK
UKHW021430280726
14060UKWH00001BA/8

9 780190 270742